The Health of Former Prisoners of War

Results from the Medical Examination Survey of Former POWs of World War II and the Korean Conflict

A Report for the Medical Follow-up Agency
Institute of Medicine

by

WILLIAM FRANK PAGE

NATIONAL ACADEMY PRESS
Washington, D.C. 1992

NATIONAL ACADEMY PRESS • 2101 Constitution Ave., N.W. • Washington, D.C. 20418

NOTICE: The project that is the subject of this report was approved by the Governing Board of the National Research Council (NRC), whose members are drawn from the councils of the National Academy of Sciences, the National Academy of Engineering, and the Institute of Medicine. Ordinarily, the NRC appoints a committee of experts to produce a report, which then undergoes independent review according to procedures approved by a Report Review Committee consisting of members of the National Academy of Sciences, the National Academy of Engineering, and the Institute of Medicine. In the case of this report, the Medical Follow-up Agency's (MFUA) general oversight body, the Committee on Epidemiology and Veterans' Follow-up Studies, has provided overall guidance; the study, however, was conducted by MFUA staff and the report written by an MFUA staff officer. Although this report has been reviewed in accordance with established NRC procedures, it represents the views of its author and not the deliberations of an expert NRC committee.

The Institute of Medicine was chartered in 1970 by the National Academy of Sciences to enlist distinguished members of the appropriate professions in the examination of policy matters pertaining to the health of the public. In this, the Institute acts under both the Academy's 1863 congressional charter responsibility to be an advisor to the federal government and its own initiative in identifying issues of medical care, research, and education.

This project was supported by funds from the Department of Veterans Affairs under contract V101(93)P-1225.

Library of Congress 92-62023
ISBN 0-309-04791-9

Additional copies of this report are available from:

National Academy Press
2101 Constitution Avenue, NW
Washington, DC 20418

B031

Printed in the United States of America

The serpent has been a symbol of long life, healing, and knowledge among almost all cultures and religions since the beginning of recorded history. The image adopted as a logotype by the Institute of Medicine is based on a relief carving from ancient Greece, now held by the Staatlichemuseen in Berlin.

Preface

The beginnings of the Medical Follow-up Agency (MFUA) study of former prisoners of war (POWs) can be found in the early 1950s when the Veterans Administration (now the Department of Veterans Affairs) initiated a program of studies of the medical status of POWs compared with non-POW controls. The latest follow-up component of this long-term study was begun in August 1986 under a contract with the National Research Council (NRC) to conduct a medical examination survey of these groups. Ordinarily, the NRC appoints a committee of experts to produce a report, which then undergoes independent review according to procedures approved by a Report Review Committee consisting of members of the National Academy of Sciences, the National Academy of Engineering, and the Institute of Medicine. In the case of this report, the MFUA's general oversight body, the Committee on Epidemiology and Veterans' Follow-up Studies—chaired by the late Richard D. Remington—has provided overall guidance; the study, however, was conducted by MFUA staff and the report written by an MFUA staff officer. Although this report has been reviewed in accordance with established NRC procedures, it represents the views of its author and not the deliberations of an expert NRC committee.

It is in the nature of long, complicated longitudinal studies such as this one that recent work builds on the foundation of earlier efforts. For that reason, I am especially appreciative of the soundness of earlier work by Cohen, Cooper, Nefzger, Beebe, and Keehn (see the reference list later in this volume). The staff of the MFUA likewise deserve acknowledgment and a great share of the credit for careful, tireless work in collecting and organizing the data on which this report is based. Special thanks go to Chiquita Benson, Harriet Crawford, and Mary Williams for their assistance.

The support of such a long, complex study—indeed, the entire series of studies—by Department of Veterans Affairs (VA) staff is also greatly appreciated. I would be remiss if I did not make special mention of project officer David Thomas and his successor, Robert Meci, as well as numerous VA Central Office staff in the Medical Research program. Space limitations prevent my thanking individually the many VA field personnel who contributed their time and experience on behalf of this study; I am particularly indebted to those VA personnel who met with me during visits to their stations. (A list of site visits can be found in Appendix B.) I would also like to thank Brian Engdahl and Steven Oboler for their helpful comments on an earlier version of this manuscript and Susan Solomon and Ellen Gerrity of the National Institute of Mental Health for their support and sponsorship of the last-minute supplemental psychological data collection.

Finally, of course, I am indebted to those former POWs and combat veterans who volunteered to come to a nearby VA medical center to be examined. Not only were the examinations themselves arduous because they were so extensive, but it was no doubt difficult to relive sometimes extraordinarily unpleasant past experiences. To our gratitude for their earlier sacrifices in wartime we must add our thanks for their recent efforts in this study.

William Frank Page

Contents

Summary

BACKGROUND

The Medical Follow-up Agency (MFUA) of the Institute of Medicine, National Academy of Sciences, conducted a medical examination survey of former prisoners of war (POWs) of World War II (WW II) and the Korean conflict. This survey, which is part of a longitudinal follow-up study begun shortly after WW II, was the first to be based on medical examinations as well as on questionnaires and records for POWs and controls. The survey focuses solely on morbidity; because no deliberate efforts were made to collect complete, cause-specific mortality data, only brief, anecdotal mortality information is presented.

PURPOSE

The goal of the research was to gather and analyze medical examination information from former POWs and comparable controls. The study design linked the MFUA's ongoing POW research and the Department of Veterans Affairs' (VA) POW protocol program to obtain information most efficiently. In brief, subjects in the MFUA study cohort were invited to a nearby VA medical center to undergo the VA protocol exam, a comprehensive physical and psychiatric examination conducted by VA medical personnel. In addition, a face-to-face psychiatric interview and a battery of psychological tests were given—to investigate the trends found in data from MFUA's 1984–1985 mail questionnaire survey on depressive symptoms.

SELECTION OF STUDY GROUPS

Because the current follow-up is grounded in earlier work, a brief summary of previous study samples is warranted; further details of the sampling plan can be found in Chapter 1 and earlier reports. For the original study samples, MFUA used the Army's official roster of all known WW II prisoners of war to select independent samples of white male Army servicemen who had been captured in the Pacific theater and the European theater (later samples of Korean conflict POWs included other races; see below). Comparable control groups were drawn from Army payroll rosters; efforts were made to balance the proportion of air and ground personnel to correspond to the composition of the POW group. Later, these original samples were augmented with several others: a group of prisoners from the European theater who were sampled from POW admissions to Army hospitals for malnutrition immediately following repatriation, a group of Korean conflict prisoners of war, and a group of comparable nonprisoner controls, selected from a file of all known U.S. Army casualties wounded in action and returned to duty in Korea. The Korean conflict POW and control groups were not limited to whites.

The current survey continues the follow-up of the same sample of POWs and controls originally assembled some 40 years ago. A total of seven study groups were investigated; their abbreviated titles and number of eligible subjects are shown below:

PWP (*P*risoners of *W*ar, *P*acific theater, WW II), 670 subjects;
WP (*W*ar veterans, *P*acific theater, WW II), 737 subjects;
PWE (*P*risoners of *W*ar, *E*uropean theater, WW II), 382 subjects;
PWEM (*P*risoners of *W*ar, *E*uropean theater, WW II, *M*alnourished), 258 subjects;
WE (*W*ar veterans, *E*uropean theater, WW II), 383 subjects;
PWK (*P*risoners of *W*ar, *K*orean conflict), 851 subjects; and
WK (*W*ar veterans, *K*orean conflict), 861 subjects.

RESEARCH QUESTIONS

The current study was charged to address the following questions.

a. Will rates of psychiatric illness, as ascertained by interview and psychological evaluation, be higher among former WW II prisoners of war of the Pacific theater (PWP) than among their nonprisoner controls? Will this also hold true for WW II prisoners of war of the European theater (PWE) and prisoners of war of the Korean conflict (PWK) when compared with their respective controls? Will rates of psychiatric illness be higher among PWP and PWK than among PWE, as observed in earlier studies?

b. What differences, if any, will there be between psychiatric illness assessed by interviewer and illness assessed by using the questionnaire? If there are differences, how will they influence the interpretation of results from (a)?

c. How have differences in illness levels changed over time? In particular, have the earlier differentials between the PWP and PWK groups, on the one hand, and the PWP and PWE groups, on the other, decreased with time?

d. How do the physical examination findings compare with the self-reported diagnoses, symptoms, and complaints from the 1984 questionnaire? Which physical findings are underreported or overreported, and how do nonmedical factors influence this reporting?

e. Is there a pattern of abnormal physical findings in the subset of PWE veterans who were seriously malnourished at repatriation?

THE IMPORTANCE OF A REPRESENTATIVE SAMPLE

Since March 1983, the Veterans Health Services and Research Administration (then the Department of Medicine and Surgery) of the VA has been conducting medical evaluations under a "POW protocol" program. The VA protocol includes a medical evaluation of standardized format, along with a standard questionnaire for collecting the POW's medical history. (This is a fairly detailed compilation of information on the POW's captivity, repatriation, and postwar adjustment.) The MFUA study was designed to use the VA's existing protocol program as the primary vehicle for data collection by simply inviting members of MFUA's longitudinal cohort to undergo a protocol examination at a nearby VA hospital. Thus, the VA's ongoing program was to do double duty—first, as an outreach program to all former POWs and second, as a data collection mechanism for a research study.

Such knowledgeable bodies as the VA's Advisory Committee on Former POWs have remarked on the value of the VA protocol exam program and the potential value of the data it collects, recommending that the information contained in the program's medical history and examination forms be made available for research use. Caution is required, however, in using these data. Although more than 30,000 examinations have been performed with the VA protocol, as a body they are limited in what they can contribute to our knowledge of POW health problems because they were gathered from a potentially biased sample about which very little is known—that is, the men who presented themselves for examination, a self-selected sample. In contrast, the members of the MFUA cohort were statistically sampled to be representative of WW II and Korean conflict POWs (and comparable veteran controls). If a large proportion of the MFUA cohort could be examined, they would presumably constitute a representative sample, the findings from which could be used to develop sound inferences and generalizations regarding the whole population of former POWs.

Mention should be made here of what might best be called the "survivor bias." Obviously, only men who survived to respond to the examination invitation could provide data for the study; presumably, less healthy men would have died earlier, and morbidity findings might thus be underrepresented. Explicit, cause-specific mortality information on this group is lacking; however, at the time of the last completed mortality follow-up in 1975, overall death rates for former POWs did not differ significantly from those of the U.S. male population of comparable age and color (i.e., white or nonwhite). Moreover, excess cause-specific mortality could be attributed to three causes: trauma, tuberculosis, and cirrhosis of the liver. In general, most of the differences between POW and general population mortality have lessened over time. Thus, there is no striking evidence from earlier mortality follow-ups that POWs die sooner than men in the general population.

RESPONSE RATES AND THE REPRESENTATIVENESS OF THE SAMPLE

Despite the careful construction of the MFUA cohort, it must be noted that its members were in a sense self-selected in that they chose to respond or not to respond to the invitation for examination. Unfortunately, response rates in the current study for both POWs and controls were very low: 40–50% among POWs and 10–14% among controls (see the findings section of this summary and also Chapter 3). However carefully the original sample was assembled, there can be no confidence with response rates as low as this that the group of respondents accurately reflects the composition of the group of all former POWs. Yet neither are such low response rates proof, in themselves, that the group of respondents is nonrepresentative. All that may rightly be said is that the statistical principles governing what one may infer from a sample—and the amount of confidence with which such inferences can be made—do not apply. A case for the representativeness of a sample based on such low response rates simply cannot be made.

Thus, the applicability of these results to the group of all POWs is unknown. There is some indication from the data comparing respondents and nonrespondents that large differences do not exist between actual respondents and all eligible subjects; nevertheless, the weight of these limited data cannot overcome the overwhelming importance of the low response rates. Consequently, the results of the study are presented as descriptive data, for two reasons.

First, even if the examination data from POWs are not strictly representative, they constitute an important case series—the largest national collection of POW examinations ever gathered together and analyzed. A number of findings in the series are worthy of note. Some confirm earlier research, and some are new; the confirmatory findings, at least, lend some weight to the validation of earlier results. New results, although they must be viewed cautiously, serve a valid scientific purpose in generating new hypotheses for more definitive studies.

The second reason to publish these data is not a scientific one. Although the report does not deal with nonscientific issues explicitly, it is recognized that the examination data will have uses beyond the scientific ones—for example, in providing material for discussion of military service–connected disabilities among former POWs. Despite the fact that sound inferences about the group of all former POWs cannot be drawn from the exam data in this report, policymakers who must deal with such issues should be able to review this descriptive information. The men who participated in these examinations also deserve an account of the process. Not to report the findings of the examination would surely raise more questions than the report, with its careful documentation of the study's limitations, would raise. The results of this examination study are thus discussed below, and we urge a maximum of reasonable caution in their interpretation and use.

METHODS

The following provides general information about the study methodology (see Chapter 2 for further details). The use of VA protocol data made it possible to perform the current study, but it also introduced several complications. Because the VA protocol examination program began before the MFUA study, a sizable proportion of the POWs in the study had been examined previously by the VA. Knowing this, study designers matched the MFUA cohort against the VA's file of completed examinations, and lists of MFUA study POWs who had already been examined were produced and sent to VA medical centers. Copies of most of these examinations have found their way to MFUA; however, the situation became more complicated when the VA asked MFUA to invite these subjects to be reexamined in order to collect additional data.

Those subjects who had not been examined previously were handled somewhat differently. First, addresses were sought for POWs in each of the three groups in the study (WW II Pacific, WW II European, and Korean conflict) and their corresponding controls. (These addresses came from the VA itself, from the Internal Revenue Service [under a special arrangement with the National Institute for Occupational Safety and Health], and from a commercial tracing firm.) Letters of invitation were mailed, as many as three per person for each of two potential addresses, urging participation in the VA medical evaluation protocol and requesting the veteran's permission to forward his name to the closest VA medical center for scheduling the examination. The VA medical centers then performed the examinations and forwarded copies of the results to MFUA. While data collection was under way in the field, MFUA staff made a number of site visits to VA medical facilities to observe the examination process.

The examination of members of the MFUA study cohort was identical to the usual VA protocol examination except that both POWs and controls underwent additional psychological testing and a more intensive psychiatric interview. The psychological testing consisted of four standardized psychological questionnaires (see Chapter 2); the usual VA psychiatric consultation, typically an unstructured part of the protocol exam, was augmented by including the posttraumatic stress disorder (PTSD) portion of the Structured Clinical Interview for DSM-III-R, Non-patient Version (SCID). These psychological tests and structured interviews provided a common framework for measuring and reporting psychological problems, which facilitated the comparison of MFUA study results with those of other research.

Toward the end of the study, it became clear that for administrative reasons, a number of examinations were being conducted without the required psychological testing. A decision was made to send blank psychological questionnaires to all potential subjects who had not completed them, regardless of examination status. Funding for this additional data collection (an initial mailing of some 2,000 questionnaires) was obtained from the National Institute of Mental Health (NIMH); the additional psychological data were added to the study's master file. A second questionnaire mailing occurred too late for its data to be included in this report.

FINDINGS

Copies of the medical examinations sent by the VA medical centers were abstracted, coded, and computerized, as were the SCID and psychological questionnaires. Unfortunately, the overall rate of completed and coded examinations was disappointingly low—as noted earlier, around 40–50% in POWs and 10–14% in controls. Some of the large apparent difference between POW and control response rates is attributable to the fact that a number of POWs came in for examinations before the formal research program began. The rate of response to the supplemental psychological questionnaire mailing sponsored by NIMH was also low: 25–30% for POWs and only 10–25% for controls. (In general, response rates among controls have been lower than those for POWs in previous morbidity follow-ups.)

The low response rates raise justifiable concerns about potential nonresponse bias, and Chapter 3 focuses on differences in demographic data for subjects who completed the entire exam and whose exams were received, abstracted, and analyzed by MFUA ("completed exams"), and all eligible subjects. Among POWs, there were no statistically significant differences between the two groups (respondents and nonrespondents) for year of birth, race, component (inductee or not), or marital status; PWP and PWK respondents, however, apparently had more education than nonrespondents, and WW II POW respondents were more apt to have served in the Army Air Corps. Data on VA hospitalization rates are displayed for three groups: subjects with completed exams, all subjects who responded to the invitation to participate (including those with completed exams), and nonrespondents. The data cover 1969–1985, predating the examination survey, and so provide evidence about differences among the three groups. There were no significant overall differences between respondents' and nonrespondents' VA hospitalization rates in any of the POW or control groups. Consequently, although the low response rates prevent any consideration of the exam data as representative, the demographic data and VA hospitalization data at least suggest that there are no overwhelming differences between respondents and nonrespondents in background characteristics or in morbidity as measured by 26 years of VA hospitalization data.

Chapter 4 of the report presents data from the 1,067 coded examinations elicited by the study. These exams provide diagnostic data on more than 65,000 coded medical conditions and are used to calculate "lifetime" prevalence rates, the probability that a given person has ever had (or still has) some specified disease, up through the time of examination. POWs were shown to have high lifetime prevalences of a number of medical conditions, but the most striking findings pertained to psychiatric illness.

Lifetime prevalence rates for selected conditions were compared with similar rates from Eberly and Engdahl's 1991 study of POW examinations at the Minneapolis VA Medical Center. The MFUA data showed elevated rates of prevalence among POWs for medical conditions related to prison camp treatment—for example, dysentery, malaria, and frozen feet—as well as for psychiatric illness. Compared with the Minneapolis POWs, the MFUA POWs had higher lifetime prevalence rates of several medical conditions, a higher rate of depressive disorder, a lower rate of PTSD, and a roughly equal rate of generalized anxiety disorder.

In Chapter 5, the discussion addresses the five basic questions listed earlier. The answer to question A, which asked whether psychiatric illness was more extensive in POWs than in controls, was that the data showed strikingly higher rates for several conditions, although no statistical tests could appropriately be applied. In particular, the rates for PTSD were appreciably higher among POWs when measured independently in each of three different ways: examination, structured clinical interview (SCID), or questionnaire (the Mississippi scale). Rates of depressive disorder were similarly elevated, again, when measured independently in three ways: examination, Center for Epidemiologic Studies depression (CES-D) questionnaire, or Beck questionnaire. The finding of a higher rate of PTSD was particularly important, given that the 1984–1985 survey had stimulated the hypothesis that PTSD was a possible psychiatric diagnosis underlying an increased rate of depressive symptoms or a comorbid condition. Additional data from the 90-item Hopkins Symptom Check List (SCL-90), however, suggested that psychiatric illness was not necessarily limited to PTSD and depressive disorder, and that there are signs of an appreciable increase in general psychopathology among POWs.

Question B asked whether there were important differences among measurement instruments for psychiatric illness. The answer for this case series was that there were appreciable differences among the various ways of measuring PTSD and depressive disorder. For PTSD, the exam and structured clinical interview—which were generally performed by the same person—agreed much more closely with each other than with the questionnaire; for depressive disorder, one scale (the CES-D) gave higher estimates of depressive disorder while the other, the Beck, gave lower estimates. Every measurement method, however, found appreciable differences between POWs and controls.

Question C asked whether earlier hospitalization rates were comparable to recent rates of self-reported hospitalization. In general, the data showed far fewer differences between POWs and controls now than in 1967. A comparison of lifetime and current prevalence rates from the current exam also showed that morbidity differences appear to have lessened over time.

Question D asked whether examination and earlier self-report questionnaire data provided comparable estimates of the prevalence of illness. Among those who completed the examinations, medical conditions were self-reported by questionnaire much less frequently than they were noted during the examination; typically, self-reported prevalence was only one-half to one-tenth the examination-based value. Some of this disparity appeared to be due to limitations in the questionnaire design (e.g., a fixed number of blanks for responses) as well as to differences between physicians and questionnaire respondents in the use of medical terminology.

Question E addressed differences between the special, albeit small, subset of severely malnourished European prisoners, PWEM, and their European theater counterparts, PWE. The case series of PWEM who were examined displayed a markedly higher lifetime prevalence of dysentery, beriberi, frozen feet, peripheral nerve disease, and gastroenteritis than was found among PWE. The latter two conditions, which were not as clearly related to war camp treatment as the others, were studied in further diagnostic detail. Excess peripheral nerve disease was attributable to excesses in three specific categories: mononeuritis of the upper limb, mononeuritis of the lower limb, and hereditary and idiopathic neuropathy. The higher prevalence of gastroenteritis was accounted for almost entirely by noninfectious gastroenteritis and colitis, rather than by irritable bowel syndrome, a disease that has already been presumptively linked to military captivity.

The analyses discussed in Chapter 5 provide evidence of psychological aftereffects of military captivity as long as 45 years after repatriation but less striking results concerning other aftereffects. Chapter 6 presents a different sort of descriptive analyses, undertaken to complement those of Chapter 5, that focused on a specific set of medical conditions taken from published reports of POW examinations at two VA medical centers, Minneapolis and Denver. Preliminary analyses of these conditions showed higher current prevalence rates among POWs for ischemic heart disease (PWEM only), peripheral nerve disease (PWP and PWK), ulcer (PWK only), gastroenteritis (PWEM and PWK), depressive disorder (PWP, PWE, PWEM, and PWK), posttraumatic stress disorder (PWP, PWEM, and PWK), and generalized anxiety disorder (PWP, PWE, PWEM, and PWK); PWP rates for malaria were appreciably *lower* than control rates. These conditions, with the exception of malaria, were included in the final stage of analysis. The entire list of selected conditions was also subjected to another set of preliminary analyses; these studies focused on determining whether the prevalence of any of the conditions was associated with the specific factors that measured harshness of treatment as a POW, such as percentage of body weight loss. All medical and psychiatric conditions with findings of either a substantially higher prevalence among some POW group or a marked association with some military captivity factor were included in the final stage of analysis.

In this stage, the prevalence data for these conditions were reanalyzed using logistic regression to determine the joint effects of weight loss and war camp symptoms, taking into account POW group differences. Prison camp symptoms were further refined into three separate measures—the presence of edema, the number of visual symptoms (such as night blindness) reported, and the number of other symptoms reported—and considered along with percent weight loss. The logistic regression analyses showed that among POWs with completed exams and earlier data on weight loss and prison camp symptoms, edema was significantly associated with a higher prevalence of ischemic heart disease and peripheral nerve disease; visual symptoms were associated with higher prevalences of cerebrovascular disease, ulcers, asthma, and PTSD; and other symptoms were associated with higher prevalences of intermittent claudication, gastroenteritis, depressive disorder, and generalized anxiety. Percent weight loss was markedly associated with a higher prevalence of intermittent claudication and arterial vascular disease and strongly associated with a *lower* prevalence of osteoarthritis. In most cases the odds ratios, which estimate the size of the increased prevalences, were between 1.0 and 2.0, indicating relatively moderate elevations in prevalence; however, the estimated effects of visual and other symptoms increased gradually with each additional reported symptom, so that the cumulative effect on the relative odds for POWs with a large number of symptoms would be quite substantial. In addition to these findings, PWP showed a higher prevalence of PTSD, compared with PWE, and among PWK, again compared with PWE, there were higher prevalences of ulcer, PTSD, schizophrenia, and generalized anxiety, as well as a *lower* prevalence of ischemic heart disease, arterial vascular disease, and asthma; these latter would appear to be age related. In general, the logistic regression analyses linking current medical conditions to earlier prison camp factors suggest more medical conditions related to the POW experience than did the simpler descriptive comparisons between POWs and controls.

After a summary of results in Chapter 7, Chapter 8 presents a detailed discussion of the study findings, comparing them with other research conducted among American and foreign POWs. In many cases, the organ-specific findings based on medical examination data were anticipated. The increased prevalence of depressive disorder, PTSD, and generalized anxiety was not unexpected, and similar findings regarding peripheral nerve disease, ulcer, and gastroenteritis likewise were not surprising. Even in these cases, however, some intriguing new data surfaced on a potential link with nutritional deficiencies, such as between ulcer and earlier visual symptoms (indicating vitamin A deficiency). The link between current peripheral nerve disease and earlier edema, indicative of a prison camp vitamin B_1 deficiency, was evidence that the well-known short-term neurological effects of (dry) beriberi are associated with persistent neurological symptoms that last for decades, even after the original nutritional disease has been successfully treated and acute symptoms have abated.

The finding of increased prevalence of schizophrenia among PWK in the case series was a new one, and a significant correlation with weight loss in this group offers material for speculation. Possible explanations include the hypothesis that organic brain syndrome arising from injury or malnutrition was incorrectly diagnosed as schizophrenia or that the association was a statistical artifact; settling the matter would require further research. Also new, and somewhat unexpected, were findings of increased asthma and cerebrovascular disease in POWs who reported visual symptoms in prison camp. Again, this involved the identification of an aftereffect of military captivity accompanied by evidence of a deficiency of vitamin A in prison camp. Findings concerning both intermittent claudication and arterial vascular disease appeared for the first time in this cohort, but their associations with percent weight loss do not provide much material to aid explanation. The last new finding, a significantly lower prevalence of osteoarthritis in POWs who reported higher weight loss in captivity, was not only unanticipated but was in the opposite direction of all other findings in Chapter 6. No explanations for it come readily to mind.

Last, but certainly not least, was the finding of a statistically significant association between ischemic heart disease and earlier reporting of localized edema. Although this finding is not exactly new, it was also not entirely expected, given that earlier studies have found conflicting evidence in both POW morbidity and mortality data. The most interesting aspect of this finding may be its specificity: localized edema was a significant risk factor for only two current medical conditions—peripheral nerve disease and ischemic heart disease—both of which were acutely related to thiamin deficiency, either the "dry" form of beriberi (peripheral nerve disease) or the "wet" form (cardiac problems). The specificity of association between localized edema and the only two medical conditions with well-established acute relationships to thiamin deficiency raises intriguing questions about the association between earlier nutritional deprivation in prison camp and subsequent chronic ischemic heart disease—even in the absence of a satisfactory explanatory biological mechanism to link the two.

In summary, excepting psychiatric illness, this report shows little evidence of widespread ill health among former prisoners of war compared with their non-POW veteran counterparts. Nevertheless, analyses of the associations between prison camp factors and subsequent disease prevalence have uncovered a number of medical conditions that can be posited as aftereffects of military captivity.

1

Background

ORIGIN AND HISTORY

The Medical Follow-up Agency (MFUA) has been studying the health of former prisoners of war (POWs) since shortly after World War II (WW II). At that time, Cohen and Cooper (1954) assembled rosters of former WW II POWs and non-POW controls and characterized their mortality, morbidity, and disability after liberation. When it began, the study differed in two important aspects from other contemporary investigations of former WW II prisoners: it was designed to study a representative sample of all former prisoners, and it included control groups. The importance of controls was emphasized by Cohen and Cooper, who asserted that "whatever the consequences of imprisonment may be, they are not likely to be grossly different in kind from the effects of combat, disease, malnutrition, and other adverse experiences encountered outside prison camps. Rather, the important effects of imprisonment will manifest themselves as differences in severity or duration, or both, so that the bases of comparison which can be provided only by suitable control groups are indispensable" (Cohen and Cooper, 1954, p. 1). The original Cohen and Cooper follow-up was also characterized by its total dependence on records—death records, hospitalization records, disability records, and questionnaires—a characteristic shared by all subsequent MFUA follow-ups.

Starting with the rosters built by Cohen and Cooper for the original study, Nefzger (1970) added Korean conflict prisoners and controls and studied the mortality of all groups. A third study, by Beebe (1975), was a

20-year morbidity follow-up, collecting data from military and Department of Veterans Affairs (then Veterans Administration; VA) records and from questionnaires. A fourth study, undertaken by Keehn (1980), continued through 1976 the mortality follow-up begun earlier. A fifth study, directed by Page (1991), was a 1984–1985 mail questionnaire follow-up that focused on the persistence of depressive symptoms. The study presented here, which was designed to collect morbidity data from 1965 through approximately 1985, also includes data collected from these earlier follow-ups. Because deliberate efforts to collect complete and detailed cause-specific mortality data were not made, only brief anecdotal mortality data are reported.

ASSEMBLY OF STUDY ROSTERS

Because this examination study followed up the MFUA cohort as assembled earlier, it is useful to review briefly the constitution of that cohort—both cases and controls. As originally constructed, the rosters of World War II ex-POWs and controls were expressly limited to white Army males, by far the largest demographically homogeneous segment of military personnel. This choice was wholly a matter of convenience "to avoid needless multiplication of variables" (Cohen and Cooper, 1954). A U.S. Army punchcard file of all prisoners liberated alive was the source of the study roster. Independent samples were drawn from the European theater of operations (which included both Mediterranean [MTO] and European [ETO] theaters); after the punchcard files were reduced to white males, sampling was carried out by selection of random digits in the service serial numbers. The samples were divided into a larger portion (group A) and a smaller (group B), with the more comprehensive morbidity follow-up performed only for group B and mortality follow-up performed for both groups A and B.

WW II controls were white Army males selected from units whose members were in combat in the theaters in which the prisoners were captured during the same time periods. Because the Pacific theater WW II prisoners were largely composed of the captured defenders of Bataan and Corregidor, and because virtually all survivors were captured, it was not possible to select controls who had contemporaneous combat service in the Pacific theater. Pacific combat controls therefore were identified from the payroll rosters of units that entered combat later. More details can be found in Cohen and Cooper (1954).

Nefzger (1970) added some Pacific prisoners to the sample, selecting them in the same way as those in the original sample except that a different combination of serial number digits was used. New controls were identified from the same payroll rosters used earlier for this study, but Nefzger matched individual controls to new prisoners on the basis of rank, arm or service, age, and race (again, all subjects were white males). Nefzger also added a new group of malnourished prisoners from the European theater, which had been derived from a 20% sample of 1945 Army hospital admissions, and a group of Korean conflict prisoners and controls selected from a file of all known U.S. Army casualties of that war. POWs were selected from a list of all repatriated prisoners, and controls were selected from the group of men who were wounded and returned to action in Korea. Thus, the Korean conflict controls differ from all other control groups because each control is the victim of a combat injury. Prisoners and controls were matched on the first digit of their Army serial number, rank, date of casualty (capture or wounding), and Army unit at the time of casualty. Selection of Korean conflict prisoners and controls was not limited in terms of race, and they were not selected to match on race; nevertheless, 85% of the former and 87% of the latter were white. Further details are available in the study report (Nefzger, 1970). Approximately 2,000 POWs from all eras and an equal number of controls were eligible for this follow-up.

Although the current survey continues the follow-up of a sample of POWs and controls originally assembled some 35 years ago, it differs from Beebe's morbidity follow-up in its inclusion of the malnourished European POWs. Thus, the survey reports data from seven study groups, shown below with the abbreviated titles that will be used in this report:

PWP (*P*risoners of *W*ar, *P*acific theater, WW II)
WP (*W*ar veterans, *P*acific theater, WW II)
PWE (*P*risoners of *W*ar, *E*uropean theater, WW II)
PWEM (*P*risoners of *W*ar, *E*uropean theater, WW II, *M*alnourished)
WE (*W*ar veterans, *E*uropean theater, WW II)
PWK (*P*risoners of *W*ar, *K*orean conflict)
WK (*W*ar veterans, *K*orean conflict).

EARLIER RESULTS

A brief discussion of the results of earlier studies provides a context for this follow-up. The earliest study, by Cohen and Cooper, found excess mortality in Pacific theater prisoners—mainly accidents and tuberculosis—but no excess mortality in European prisoners. It also identified tuberculosis, residual effects of malnutrition, psychological problems, ophthalmic changes, gastrointestinal disorders, and cardiovascular disease as frequent conditions worthy of continued study. Nefzger's mortality follow-up showed that the early excess mortality had begun to diminish by the mid-1960s among WW II POWs, while Korean conflict former POWs continued to have higher mortality throughout the entire 12 years of follow-up in that study. Beebe, in a 1965 questionnaire and record follow-up, noted that

Pacific WW II prisoners were experiencing both somatic and psychological aftereffects, whereas European prisoners apparently were experiencing only psychological aftereffects. Higher rates of illness were manifested in higher hospitalization rates, higher VA disability compensation rates, and more self-reported health problems. Keehn's mortality follow-up through the mid-1970s documented the fact that the increased early risk of dying among WW II Pacific and Korean conflict prisoners had lessened over time. In fact, for these POWs, as well as for the WW II European POWs, overall death rates in the most recent follow-up period were indistinguishable from those of the comparably aged U.S. population.

Particularly important to the current study are the results of the latest completed follow-up, a 1984–1985 mail questionnaire survey. This follow-up found that detrimental psychological effects of military captivity persisted for as long as 40 years after repatriation. (Beebe had shown earlier that 20 years after repatriation, the most striking and persistent aftereffects of the POW experience were psychological.) The 1984–1985 follow-up collected data on depressive symptoms, as measured by the Center for Epidemiologic Studies depression (CES-D) scale developed at the National Institute of Mental Health; it found rates of depressive symptoms among POWs that were from three to five times higher than expected from comparable studies of the general population. Equally important, the follow-up showed that depressive symptoms were more severe among POWs who had been treated more harshly during captivity, although POWs who were older at capture and who had more education had less depressive symptomatology than younger, less well-educated POWs. It was speculated, however, that these findings on depressive symptoms were actually due to a higher prevalence of some underlying diagnosis, probably posttraumatic stress disorder.

The design of the current study drew on these earlier follow-ups in deciding on the basic kinds of data that should be collected. First, it was clearly time for a more general morbidity survey; using VA medical practitioners to collect data as part of a comprehensive medical examination would provide the first such examination data since repatriation, as well as the most complete morbidity information since Beebe's follow-up study in 1967. Second, the 1984–1985 results pointed out the need to obtain diagnostic data from physicians as well as self-reported symptom data. Thus, the current study consisted of a comprehensive medical examination, to achieve the first objective, plus a structured clinical interview and comprehensive psychiatric evaluation, to achieve the second.

REFERENCES

Beebe GW. 1975. Follow-up studies of World War II and Korean war prisoners: II. Morbidity, disability, and maladjustments. Am. J. Epidemiol. 101:400-422.

Cohen BM, Cooper MZ. 1954. A Follow-up Study of World War II Prisoners of War. Veterans Administration Medical Monograph. Government Printing Office, Washington, DC.

Keehn RJ. 1980. Follow-up studies of World War II and Korean war prisoners. III. Mortality to January 1, 1976. Am. J. Epidemiol. 111:194-211.

Nefzger MD. 1970. Follow-up studies of World War II and Korean war prisoners. I. Study plan and mortality findings. Am. J. Epidemiol. 91:123-138.

Page WF, Engdahl BE, Eberly RE. 1991. Prevalence and correlates of depressive symptoms among former prisoners of war. J. Nerv. Ment. Dis. 179:670-677.

2

Data Collection Procedures

The current MFUA study is the sixth such study of the group of POWs and controls assembled some four decades ago. Previous efforts have focused on mortality, as ascertained from death certificates, and on morbidity, as reported in VA records and in questionnaires mailed to study subjects. The data for the current study are unique: both former POWs and veteran controls were invited to undergo a comprehensive medical and mental health examination at a nearby VA medical facility; the results of the examination were sent to MFUA for analysis.

This approach took advantage of the ongoing POW examination program, called the POW Protocol Examination program, that was already in place in VA medical facilities when this research began. Because of the existing program, MFUA collected its research examination data by inviting study subjects to participate in the VA program and then receiving a copy of the VA examination results. In order to include the MFUA research subjects in the VA program, it was necessary for the VA Central Office to issue a circular to its field stations, directing them to perform these examinations and send copies to MFUA. Because of administrative procedures, there were at one time two VA circulars in the field (one for POW examinations and one for control examinations); copies of these circulars can be found in Appendix A.

Although the overall study design was quite straightforward, a complicating factor arose in the form of potential study subjects who had already been examined under the VA program for their own personal reasons. Originally, these subjects, called "volunteers," were not asked to undergo a reexamination but instead were identified by matching them against the VA POW exam tracking system, which contains a record for each POW who has undergone the VA's protocol exam. Requests for their already completed examinations were then sent directly to the VA field stations. (More details about this process are provided later in this chapter.)

The issue of volunteers became somewhat more complicated, however, when a site visit by a VA team in August 1989 resulted in a recommendation that volunteers be reexamined. As a result, volunteers were mailed invitations and processed similarly to study subjects who had not been previously examined. The only remaining complication was the possibility that MFUA might receive reports of two examinations for an individual—one done before its invitation and one done afterward. In such cases, only the most recent exam was included in the analyses.

If a study subject had not undergone a POW protocol examination (or later, after volunteers were solicited, even if he had), an invitation was issued by MFUA for the man to undergo examination at a nearby VA hospital. Using addresses on file from previous MFUA follow-up studies or addresses obtained from the VA, the Internal Revenue Service, or a commercial tracing firm (Equifax), MFUA staff mailed subjects as many as three invitations, each of them tracked by a computerized mailing system. If a new address was obtained at any time during the study, fourth, fifth, and sixth mailings were attempted if needed.

Once a study subject agreed to be examined, this fact was logged into the mailing system and used to produce a list of subjects to be scheduled for examination at each VA hospital. Over the course of the study, more than a dozen such schedule lists were sent to VA medical facilities. When the examinations were completed, copies were sent to MFUA, which were then sent out to be abstracted, coded, and computerized by trained nosologists under MFUA's contract with GRG Associates, a local subcontractor.

DETAILS OF THE DATA COLLECTION PROCESS

Much of the invitation letter process was automated, and a computerized mail system developed in an earlier POW study was used to generate and print mailing labels and keep track of mailing dates and mail status information. The complete mail package included a cover letter, a postage-paid envelope, and a response form on which the subject indicated his willingness to participate and provided contacting information, such as his home or work telephone number (see Appendix A).

When responses were received from the mailing, they were logged into the mailing system. In most cases the response (or lack of it) was easy to categorize, and the following codes were simply entered into the system:

1 = invitation returned, agreed to participate
2 = RWA (returned without address)
3 = refusal, do not mail again
4 = invitation returned marked deceased, death not verified
5 = deceased, verified; do not mail again
6 = unable to participate
7 = previously examined
A = subject claims he was already examined
R = recontact veteran to clarify exam status
V = volunteer (this code was only assigned before mailing).

Some discussion is necessary regarding a few of these codes. An unverified death (code 4) was one for which MFUA received notice but no official record, such as a death certificate. "Unable to participate" (code 6) was differentiated from refusal by the subject's indicating a willingness to be examined but his also citing conditions such as poor health or long distances that made his participation difficult or impossible. Code A was assigned when a subject claimed a previous examination even though he had not been identified as a volunteer. In such instances, MFUA attempted to contact the VA hospital to obtain a copy of this exam. If no examination was available, the mail system code was changed to R (recontact), and another letter was sent. Code R was also used in cases in which, for example, the subject returned the response form but failed to check the box indicating his willingness to participate. Any address changes noted on the response form were also logged into the mail system upon return.

At the same time that examination requests were being sent to individuals, requests were being sent to VA hospitals for copies of already completed exams undergone by the "volunteers." To accomplish this, lists of subjects who were thought to have undergone examination were sent to VA medical facilities. In this request for information, as with the previously described schedule list, two identical copies of the letter and list were sent to the facilities from which completed exams were requested: one copy went to the POW administrative coordinator and one to the physician coordinator. (Every VA medical facility that performs POW examinations has both a physician coordinator and an administrative coordinator.) Requests for completed examinations were made periodically.

After a subject had indicated an interest in being examined, it was necessary to notify a nearby VA medical center of his interest. Each such subject was first assigned to the nearest VA medical facility, gauging distances by road atlas. There was also an attempt to assign the subject to a VA hospital based on VA-defined catchment areas, but there were some cases in which the VA facility determined by catchment area would not have been the one closest to the subject. In other cases, the respondent may have indicated a preferred VA facility, which was almost always honored.

Once the hospital assignment had been made, the schedule lists were produced automatically at specified times, each containing the names and identifying numbers of the study subjects to be examined. Transmitted with the schedule list was the original response form for each person on the list, accompanied by a cover letter. The computerized mail system tracked the status of each exam request by individual subject.

Before contacting a subject for examination, however, each VA hospital involved in the study was required to make arrangements for review of the study protocol by the appropriate local review committee that dealt with human subjects research. Although a study protocol and sample informed consent document were included in the VA circulars guiding the study, each hospital was responsible for securing the approval of its local committee before undertaking data collection.

When the completed examinations were returned, they were first carefully separated, checked, and logged in. The complete examination package was supposed to include all of the following: a *POW medical history form* (VA Form 10-0048); a *summary sheet* containing the final list of diagnoses, prepared by the POW physician after all laboratory results and consultations were received; a *physician's history and physical*; a *social work consultation* (sometimes called a psychosocial history); a *mental health evaluation* (either a psychological or psychiatric consultation), which was supposed to include the *posttraumatic stress disorder (PTSD) portion of the Structured Clinical Interview for the third revised edition of the Diagnostic and Statistical Manual (DSM-III-R)*; and finally the *four psychological questionnaires*, known as forms A (the Beck depression scale), B (the Center for Epidemiologic Studies depression [CES-D] scale), C (the 90-item Hopkins symptom checklist [SCL-90]), and D (the Mississippi PTSD scale). Incomplete examinations were noted in a separate file, and attempts were made later to contact the VA hospitals and obtain these missing pieces.

Because the research exams included additional items such as the structured clinical interview for PTSD and the psychological questionnaires, a brief discussion of these items is warranted. An abbreviated version of the Structured Clinical Interview for DSM-III-R, Non-patient Version (Spitzer et al., 1986), hereafter SCID, was used in this study because it was felt that the full-length SCID—some 90 pages long—could not be successfully administered. Given the potential importance of PTSD among POWs and the need to keep short any additional data collection demands, only the 8-page PTSD portion of the SCID was chosen for inclusion in the exam; in order to use this form, references to Vietnam service were removed to make it applicable to POWs and controls from WW II and the Korean conflict. Although no special training was given to field personnel regarding the SCID, instructions concerning its administration were included in the directives (i.e., VA circulars) sent to all VA facilities; there were no explicit attempts to assess interrater reliability. The PTSD portion of the SCID is designed in such a way as to allow the interviewer independently to record information pertinent to both lifetime and current symptoms of PTSD. The interviewer then provides his or her separate assessments of these diagnoses. In general, the same person who performed the mental status examination also administered the SCID.

The four psychological questionnaires were standard instruments, each of which was chosen for different purposes. The CES-D (Radloff, 1977) was an obvious choice, given its use in the 1984–1985 follow-up, and offered the additional advantage of obtaining test–retest data. The Beck depression scale (Beck et al., 1961) was chosen because it is more widely known and accepted in clinical circles than the CES-D, which has been used more in epidemiologic and general population studies. The Mississippi PTSD scale (Keane et al., 1984) is a paper-and-pencil test originally developed to measure the presence of PTSD in populations of Vietnam veterans. The SCL-90 (Derogatis et al., 1973) is a widely used general checklist of psychological symptoms. In all cases, standard scoring of these instruments was done, and well-established "cut-off" scores were used: for the CES-D scale, a score of 16 or more being evidence of depressive symptoms; for the Beck scale, less than 10 indicating no evidence of depression; 10–18, evidence of mild depression; 19–29, evidence of moderate depression; and 30 or more, evidence of marked depression. For the 35-item Mississippi scale, 89 or more was evidence of PTSD (Kulka et al., 1991).

The status of every exam received was tracked by the computerized mail system. Complete and incomplete exams were simply coded C and I, respectively, but in some instances other status codes were assigned based on information received from the VA hospital if, for example, the exam itself could not be completed. The following codes were provided only by VA hospitals on returned schedule lists and were entered directly into the exam status field:

1 = exam scheduled
2 = exam previously done—do not repeat if exam was complete
3 = VA unable to contact
4 = subject refused examination (at the VA hospital)
5 = subject physically unable to come for exam
6 = subject deceased (reported by VA hospital)
7 = VA hospital able to contact but subject moved out of area.

Three additional codes—U, N, and G—were infrequently entered. Code U was assigned when the VA hospital was unable to locate an examination that had supposedly been completed; code N was given when there was no exam done on a volunteer; and code G was used when the medical facility suggested that MFUA request the subject's VA claims folder (a "form G" request) to obtain a copy of the exam.

In some cases, MFUA found that an exam had been transferred from one VA hospital to another, which usually happened when a veteran found that another VA facility was more convenient than the one MFUA had assigned. The computerized mail system, which allowed up to three VA medical facilities to be entered onto the file, was used to track such transfers. The contract with the VA did not provide for payment of research subjects for their participation in the study. It did, however, allow MFUA to reimburse participants directly for their mileage expenses at a slightly higher rate than permitted by local VA facilities.

The abstracting, coding, and computerization of completed examinations was done by a subcontractor, GRG Associates. Examinations were generally sent in batches of 50, and each batch of completed exams was returned along with a floppy disk containing the abstracted information and a hard-copy printout of the abstracted and coded information. All medical conditions noted in the examination were coded by a trained nosologist using the ninth edition of the International Classification of Diseases, Clinical Modification (ICD-9-CM).

Each coded condition was also categorized as to its source within the examination: discharge summary; history; findings; laboratory, x-ray, or other such services; psychiatric or psychological consultation; medical consultation; or VA benefits application form. Thus, a specific condition might appear several times, with different sources, in a single coded record. Data on the resolution of each medical condition were also provided by the coder, based on available material in the exam (e.g., whether the subject was still under treatment, still receiving medication, no longer had a problem, etc.). If there was no information about a condition being resolved, it was considered unresolved. Data on medications were also recorded exactly as noted in the record, and each recorded medication was associated with a particular diagnosis; these recorded data, however, were not edited or abstracted further and so are not included in the analyses of this report. In each batch, a sample of hard-copy abstracts was spot-checked against the original examinations. If an unusually high number of errors were detected, that batch was sent back to GRG for correction.

The POW medical history forms (VA Forms 10-0048) were keyed by MFUA personnel into a separate data file, as were the SCID and psychological test forms. A random sample of medical history forms was printed and checked by hand against the original forms.

Toward the end of the study, it became clear that the number of completed exams would be much greater than the number of completed psychological questionnaires, in part because volunteers who were not reexamined did not get a chance to fill out the psychological questionnaires. It was decided to address a last-minute, separate direct mailing to study subjects to request the psychological questionnaire data. With the sponsorship of the

National Institute of Mental Health, MFUA mailed some 2,000 questionnaires to POWs and controls who were not known to be dead, who had a valid mailing address, and who had no psychological questionnaires on file. When returned, these questionnaires were keyed and added to the data file for analysis. A second mailing was made to nonrespondents, but these data were available too late for inclusion in this report.

The next chapter reviews the final status of data collection, with a focus on the response rates for the medical examination and for the psychological questionnaires.

REFERENCES

Beck AT, Ward CH, Mendelson M, et al. 1961. An inventory for measuring depression. Arch. Gen. Psychiatr. 4:561-571.

Derogatis LR, Lipman RS, Covi L. 1973. The SCL-90: an outpatient psychiatric rating scale. Psychopharmacol. Bull. 9:13-28.

Keane TM, Malloy PF, Fairbank JA. 1984. Empirical development of an MMPI subscale for the assessment of combat-related posttraumatic stress disorder. J. Consult. Clin. Psychol. 52:888-891.

Kulka RA, Schlenger WE, Fairbank JA, et al. 1991. Assessment of posttraumatic stress disorder in the community: prospects and pitfalls from recent studies of Vietnam veterans. Psychol. Assess. 3:547-560.

Radloff LS. 1977. The CES-D scale: a self-report depression scale for research in the general population. Appl. Psychol. Meas. I:385-401.

Spitzer RL, William JB, Gibbon M. 1986. Structured Clinical Interview for DSM-III, Non-patient version (SCID-NP-V; 12/1/86). Biometrics Research Department, New York State Psychiatric Institute. New York, NY.

3

Final Status of Data Collection

The current study of the MFUA cohort of former POWs and veteran controls differs substantially from earlier efforts in that it collected data by examination rather than by mail questionnaire or record review. Response rates for the examination were disappointingly low—much lower than response rates for earlier follow-up efforts—which calls into question the representativeness of the participating group. This chapter examines in detail invitation rates, response rates, and the issue of representativeness.

Table 3.1 shows invitation and response rates by group for POWs and controls. The first appreciable difference between POWs and their corresponding controls is in their invitation rates. Despite the fact that addresses were sought from a number of independent sources, such as the Internal Revenue Service, the VA, and a commercial tracing firm (see Chapter 2 for details), address-finding was much more successful for the study's POWs than for its controls. In particular, invitations were issued to 95% or more of POWs (the PWEM group was the exception at 86%) versus roughly 75% of controls; the WK group was somewhat higher at 87%. Most of this difference between POW and control invitation rates is attributable to the design of previous follow-up efforts. The latest completed follow-up in 1984–1985 included all POW groups but only the WK controls. Because WW II controls had not been traced since 1965, their current addresses were more difficult to obtain, and in consequence their invitation rates were lower. Moreover, a high proportion of former POWs (as well as the WK controls) receive VA disability compensation and are more likely to be successfully traced using VA records.

TABLE 3.1 Invitation and Response Rates (numbers and percentages[a]) for the Medical Examination, by Study Group

Item	PWP	PWE	PWEM	PWK	WP	WE	WK
Number of eligible subjects at start of study	670 (100.0)	382 (100.0)	258 (100.0)	851 (100.0)	737 (100.0)	383 (100.0)	861 (100.0)
Number of invitations mailed	650 (97.0)	367 (96.1)	222 (86.0)	805 (94.6)	551 (74.8)	302 (78.9)	751 (87.2)
Responses to mailing							
Agreed	210 (32.3)	153 (41.6)	76 (34.2)	340 (42.2)	145 (26.3)	69 (22.8)	294 (39.1)
Refused	132 (20.3)	83 (22.7)	43 (19.4)	123 (15.3)	110 (20.0)	68 (22.5)	160 (21.3)
No response	88 (13.5)	53 (14.4)	43 (19.4)	149 (18.5)	147 (26.7)	85 (28.1)	212 (28.2)
Previous exam	92 (14.2)	20 (5.4)	19 (8.6)	126 (15.7)	—	—	—
Dead[b]	128 (19.7)	58 (15.8)	41 (18.5)	67 (8.3)	149 (27.0)	80 (26.5)	85 (11.3)
Number of exams completed[b]	250 (38.5)	142 (38.7)	83 (37.4)	408 (50.7)	54 (9.8)	27 (8.9)	103 (13.7)

PWP, prisoner of war, Pacific theater, WW II; PWE, prisoner of war, European theater, WW II; PWEM, prisoner of war, malnourished, European theater, WW II; PWK, prisoner of war, Korean conflict; WP, war veteran, Pacific theater, WW II; WE, war veteran, European theater, WW II; WK, wounded war veteran, Korean conflict.

[a]Percentages appear in parentheses.

[b]For POWs only, subjects who died but who had provided a completed examination before their death are included in the number and percentage of completed calculations.

TABLE 3.2 Invitation and Response Rates (numbers and percentages[a]) for the Psychological Questionnaire, by Study Group

Item	PWP	PWE	PWEM	PWK	WP	WE	WK
Number of eligible subjects at start of study	670	382	258	851	737	383	861
Number who returned a questionnaire at exam	42	34	16	99	24	10	43
Number who were mailed a questionnaire[b]	316 (100.0)	193 (100.0)	115 (100.0)	484 (100.0)	270 (100.0)	142 (100.0)	464 (100.0)
Responses to mailing							
Returned questionnaire	130 (41.1)	86 (44.6)	46 (40.0)	169 (34.9)	71 (26.3)	30 (21.1)	142 (30.6)
No response	164 (51.9)	92 (47.7)	64 (55.7)	258 (53.3)	183 (67.8)	104 (73.2)	291 (62.7)
Dead	7 (2.3)	3 (1.6)	2 (1.7)	6 (1.2)	3 (1.1)	2 (1.4)	4 (0.8)
Returned, wrong address	15 (4.7)	12 (6.2)	3 (2.6)	19 (3.9)	13 (4.8)	6 (4.2)	27 (5.8)
Total questionnaires received[c]	172 (25.7)	120 (31.4)	60 (23.3)	268 (31.5)	95 (12.9)	40 (10.4)	185 (21.5)

PWP, prisoner of war, Pacific theater, WW II; PWE, prisoner of war, European theater, WW II; PWEM, prisoner of war, malnourished, European theater, WW II; PWK, prisoner of war, Korean conflict; WP, war veteran, Pacific theater, WW II; WE, war veteran, European theater, WW II; WK, wounded war veteran, Korean conflict.

[a]Percentages appear in parentheses.

[b]Excludes those who turned in a questionnaire at their examination, those who refused further contact, those who were identified as deceased during examination invitation, and those without a good mailing address.

[c]Including the second mailing responses, through June 1, 1992, yields the following: PWP 211 (31.5%); PWE 144 (37.7%); PWEM 75 (29.1%); PWK 317 (37.3%); WP 114 (15.5%); WE 49 (12.8%); and WK 222 (25.8%).

Limiting the remaining discussion to invited subjects only, one sees that POW agreement rates are higher and their refusal and no-response rates lower than those of controls. The interpretation of this differential response, however, is complicated by the fact that all POW groups included so-called "volunteers" (see Chapter 2), that is, those POWs who had come in for examination before the start of MFUA's follow-up. These POWs thus may have provided information to the study even if they subsequently refused an invitation for a reexamination or died. It must also be emphasized that the death information reported in Table 3.1 was obtained mainly as a result of unverified notification of deaths by next of kin; these data cannot be considered accurate or complete enough to permit the calculation of even crude mortality rates.

The rates of completed examinations, shown on the bottom of Table 3.1, are the most important figures in the table. They show that examination data were available for 38–50% of eligible (invited) POWs, a rate substantially higher than that of controls, of whom only 8–14% provided examination data. Such a disparity raises the obvious issue of potential nonresponse bias, which is addressed later in this chapter. However, if subjects who died were eliminated as ineligible from the control groups—a reasonable action because deceased controls, unlike deceased POW volunteers, could not possibly have provided any examination information—this marginally raises the proportion of completed examinations to 11.3% for WE, 16.1% for WK, and 13.3% for WP.

As mentioned in Chapter 2, supplemental funding from the National Institute of Mental Health enabled a last-minute collection of psychiatric data by mail questionnaire. The process of contacting study subjects directly and having them mail in their psychological questionnaires, rather than waiting for these data to come in with the medical examination, resulted in a notably higher number of responses. Questionnaires that arrived in response to the second mailing, however, came too late to be included in the analyses for this report. Hence, the response rates seen in Table 3.2 reflect only responses to the first mailing.

Table 3.2 shows that POW response rates to the questionnaire were between 35% and 40%, higher than the 20–30% response rates for controls. Adding in those psychological questionnaires that were returned at the time of the exam yields total questionnaire response rates of 26–32% for POWs and 10–28% for controls. It is noteworthy that WK had the highest total response rate of all control groups, even higher than PWP.

The low response rates observed for both POWs and controls mean that, no matter how carefully the original sample was constructed, there can be no confidence that the group of respondents accurately reflects the composition of the entire group of POWs and controls. To be fair, low response rates do not, in themselves, prove that the group of respondents is nonrepre-

TABLE 3.3 Demographic Characteristics Before Capture[a] for Examination Respondents and All Eligible Subjects, by Study Group (percentages in parentheses[b])

Demographic Characteristic	PWP Exam	PWP No Exam	PWE Exam	PWE No Exam	PWK Exam	PWK No Exam	WP Exam	WP No Exam	WE Exam	WE No Exam	WK Exam	WK No Exam
Year of Birth												
<1910	8	29	3	5	1	1	0	29	1	11	0	3
	(3.2)	(6.9)	(2.1)	(2.1)	(0.2)	(0.2)	(0.0)	(4.2)	(3.7)	(3.1)	(0.0)	(0.4)
1910–1919	147	257	56	98	13	36	36	448	12	162	8	44
	(58.8)	(61.2)	(39.4)	(40.8)	(3.2)	(8.1)	(66.7)	(65.6)	(44.4)	(45.1)	(7.8)	(5.8)
1920–1929	95	134	83	137	203	202	17	207	12	185	51	374
	(38.0)	(31.9)	(58.5)	(57.1)	(49.8)	(45.6)	(31.5)	(30.3)	(44.4)	(51.5)	(49.5)	(49.3)
1930–	—	—	—	—	191	204	—	—	—	—	43	338
	—	—	—	—	(46.8)	(46.0)	—	—	—	—	(41.7)	(44.5)
Race												
White	249	419	141	240	356	376	54	680	24	358	93	661
	(99.6)	(99.8)	(99.3)	(100.0)	(87.3)	(84.9)	(100.0)	(99.6)	(88.9)	(99.7)	(90.3)	(87.1)
Black	—	—	—	—	33	48	—	—	—	—	7	71
	—	—	—	—	(8.1)	(10.8)	—	—	—	—	(6.8)	(9.4)
Other	—	—	—	—	19	18	—	—	—	—	2	25
	—	—	—	—	(4.7)	(4.1)	—	—	—	—	(1.9)	(3.3)
Component												
Inductee	34	79	104	175	114	124	19	244	11	256	30	198
	(13.6)	(18.8)	(73.2)	(72.9)	(27.0)	(28.0)	(35.2)	(35.7)	(40.7)	(71.3)	(29.1)	(26.1)
Other	213	339	37	65	294	319	35	436	13	102	72	561
	(85.2)	(80.7)	(26.1)	(27.1)	(72.1)	(72.0)	(64.8)	(63.8)	(48.1)	(28.4)	(69.9)	(73.0)

Marital status												
Single	231	391	118	187	348	377	44	615	23	283	85	634
	(92.4)	(93.1)	(83.1)	(77.9)	(85.3)	(85.1)	(81.5)	(90.0)	(85.2)	(78.8)	(82.5)	(83.5)
Other	18	27	24	53	59	62	9	63	1	74	17	121
	(7.2)	(6.4)	(16.9)	(22.1)	(14.5)	(14.0)	(16.7)	(9.2)	(3.7)	(20.6)	(16.5)	(15.9)
Years of education												
0–8	38	100	29	48	149	163	10	166	4	92	38	252
	(15.2)	(23.8)	(20.4)	(20.0)	(36.5)	(36.8)	(18.5)	(24.3)	(14.8)	(25.6)	(36.9)	(33.2)
9–11	70	134	29	69	154	201	12	212	4	83	31	326
	(28.0)	(31.9)	(20.4)	(28.8)	(37.7)	(45.4)	(22.2)	(31.0)	(14.8)	(23.1)	(30.1)	(43.0)
12	87	118	54	88	84	59	20	195	8	107	25	131
	(34.8)	(28.1)	(38.0)	(36.7)	(20.6)	(13.3)	(37.0)	(28.6)	(29.6)	(29.8)	(24.3)	(17.3)
≥13	54	69	30	34	21	17	11	106	8	75	8	49
	(21.6)	(16.4)	(21.1)	(14.2)	(5.1)	(3.8)	(20.4)	(15.5)	(29.7)	(20.9)	(7.8)	(6.5)
Arm or service at selection												
Arms	115	226	57	130	363	402	33	392	10	214	93	705
	(46.0)	(53.8)	(40.1)	(54.2)	(89.0)	(90.7)	(61.1)	(57.4)	(37.0)	(59.6)	(90.3)	(92.9)
Technical	39	82	12	25	44	41	5	108	0	1	9	51
	(15.6)	(19.5)	(8.5)	(10.4)	(10.8)	(9.3)	(9.3)	(15.8)	(0.0)	(0.3)	(8.7)	(6.7)
Air Corps	96	111	73	85	—	—	16	180	14	143	—	—
	(38.4)	(26.4)	(51.4)	(35.4)	—	—	(29.6)	(26.4)	(51.9)	(39.8)	—	—
Total[c]	420	250	240	142	443	408	683	54	359	27	759	103

PWP, prisoner of war, Pacific theater, WW II; PWE, prisoner of war, European theater, WW II; PWK, prisoner of war, Korean conflict; WP, war veteran, Pacific theater, WW II; WE, war veteran, European theater, WW II; WK, wounded war veteran, Korean conflict.

[a]Control date equivalent to POW capture date.
[b]Percentages appear in parentheses.
[c]The counts for subgroups may not match the totals because unknowns are omitted.

sentative. However, the statistical principles that determine how inferences may be drawn from statistical samples do not apply when response rates are as low as they are in this instance. Consequently, a case for the representativeness of the group of respondents simply cannot be made.

Nevertheless, it is still worthwhile to examine the actual composition of the group of respondents and compare it with that of the original sample to determine how unrepresentative it appears to be. There are two kinds of data available for comparison: demographic and hospitalization data.

Demographic data were gathered from military records and are available from virtually the entire sample. Table 3.3 shows demographic data by POW and control study group, comparing those having completed examinations with all subjects eligible for the study. There were relatively few differences between subjects with completed examinations and all eligible subjects. Among WW II POWs, there were appreciably higher proportions of men with service in the Army Air Corps—servicemen who were captured when their planes were shot down were held as POWs; among the PWP and PWK groups, respondents had notably higher levels of education. In the WE group, compared with other controls, there was a higher proportion of examined men who were single at the time of entry into service or who were inductees. The usual kinds of statistical tests of differences are not appropriate here, because such tests focus on the effects of sampling error (i.e., the specific error that would arise from having examined only a sample and not the whole group of either POWs or controls); with such low response rates, there is the clear potential for large, unmeasurable errors due to nonresponse.

Not all demographic characteristics of possible interest were, or could be, examined. Factors such as the distance of a subject from the nearest VA medical facility, for example, were applicable only to those who came to the examination and were reimbursed for travel expenses by MFUA. Of course, not even a complete examination of all available demographic data and a finding of few or no differences would provide appropriate, sufficient evidence to conclude that a group of respondents is a representative sample. Nevertheless, based on an examination of these selected demographic characteristics, there is little evidence to suggest that the group of respondents differs substantially from nonrespondents.

The comparison hospital data also provide additional evidence that responders and nonresponders are not radically different. Prior to the beginning of the examination study, data were obtained on VA hospitalizations from 1969 to 1985 for all of the study's eligible subjects. Table 3.4 shows VA hospitalization rates for those with completed exams, for eligible nonrespondents, and for ineligible subjects. (The latter are those to whom invitations were not mailed or who were discovered to be deceased.)

The most important comparison in Table 3.4 is between subjects with completed exams (respondents) and those eligible to be examined who did not provide exam data (nonrespondents). In most cases, the two VA hospitalization rates are fairly similar across the POW and control groups. There are some differences—particularly in the Pacific theater WW II groups—but interestingly the direction of these differences is not uniform across all study groups. Subjects with completed examinations had higher VA hospitalization rates in the PWE, PWEM, WP, and WK groups; subjects with completed exams in the WE, PWP, and PWK groups had lower VA hospitalization rates. With the exception of the WP group, ineligible subjects had the highest VA hospitalization rates, presumably because that group included deceased subjects who might be expected to have higher VA hospitalization rates.

These findings are further concrete, if only partial, evidence that differences identified in the health of respondents and nonrespondents were relatively small; indeed, similar evidence was adduced by Beebe (1975) in his 1967 morbidity follow-up study. Along the same lines, Page (1991) estimated the effects of nonresponse in the 1984–1985 questionnaire follow-up and found no evidence of any appreciable bias. Sample sizes in Table 3.4 are nonetheless quite small, especially in the control groups, and the WP group is unusual in the large difference in hospitalization rates between respondents and nonrespondents and in the fact that respondents had higher

TABLE 3.4 Comparison of VA Hospitalization Rates for Examination Study Respondents and Nonrespondents, by Study Group (average ± standard error, *N* in parentheses)

	Type of Respondent		
Study Group	Exam Completed	Eligible, Exam Not Completed	Not Eligible[a]
PWE	0.338 ± 0.088 (142)	0.244 ± 0.067 (176)	0.547 ± 0.167 (64)
PWEM	0.627 ± 0.180 (83)	0.421 ± 0.118 (107)	0.705 ± 0.203 (68)
WE	0.160 ± 0.095 (25)	0.228 ± 0.069 (197)	0.783 ± 0.147 (161)
PWP	0.892 ± 0.105 (250)	1.058 ± 0.111 (293)	1.520 ± 0.201 (127)
WP	0.778 ± 0.230 (54)	0.342 ± 0.060 (348)	0.411 ± 0.073 (335)
PWK	0.745 ± 0.074 (408)	0.799 ± 0.093 (338)	1.143 ± 0.209 (105)
WK	0.422 ± 0.119 (102)	0.387 ± 0.047 (564)	0.610 ± 0.112 (195)

PWP, prisoner of war, Pacific theater, WW II; PWE, prisoner of war, European theater, WW II; PWEM, prisoner of war, malnourished, European theater, WW II; PWK, prisoner of war, Korean conflict; WP, war veteran, Pacific theater, WW II; WE, war veteran, European theater, WW II; WK, wounded war veteran, Korean conflict.

[a]Unverified death, invitation never mailed, or invitation returned because of wrong address.

VA hospitalization rates than ineligibles. While not entirely comforting, the data in Table 3.4 do suggest that nonresponse bias is not overwhelmingly large, although it cannot be asserted that VA hospitalization rates are the most appropriate way to gauge overall health.

Because the low response rates for POWs and controls vitiate any arguments about the representativeness of the groups of POW or control examinees, the examinations that were collected must be considered case study material and the analyses in the remainder of this report purely descriptive. With this understanding, the report moves next to further discussion in Chapter 4 of the examination format and details of data collection, along with the presentation of some preliminary results and comparisons with the results of another VA exam–based study. After this, the principal study questions will be taken up in Chapter 5.

REFERENCES

Beebe GW. 1975. Follow-up studies of World War II and Korean war prisoners. II. Morbidity, disability, and maladjustments. Am. J. Epidemiol. 101:400-422.

Page WF. 1991. Using longitudinal data to estimate nonresponse bias. Soc. Psychiatry Psychiatr. Epidemiol. 26:127-131.

4

General Results

This chapter presents a brief introduction to the examination data, beginning with a more detailed discussion of their collection, coding, and organization. As stated in Chapter 2, all examination data were abstracted and coded by trained nosologists using ninth edition International Classification of Diseases, Clinical Modification (ICD-9-CM) codes. Additionally, they recorded the source of each coded medical condition within the exam as one of the following: discharge summary; history; findings; laboratory, x-ray, or other such services; psychiatric or psychological examination; medical consultation; or VA benefits application form. Medical conditions were also characterized as to their time of onset (while a prisoner of war or not, for example) and whether they were currently resolved. Medications being taken for a given condition were also abstracted and keyed, but the complexity and the lack of standardization of these data prevented their analysis and inclusion in this report.

The additional coding of the source and resolution of each medical condition was undertaken to provide information that might help account for some of the variability in the exams themselves. Although the VA circulars provided directives about the general scope of the exam, the conduct of the exam varied from facility to facility largely because of differences among examiners in the performance of the comprehensive medical examination. Moreover, there were some additional administrative differences among examination sites that contributed to examination variability—for example, the number of days it took to conduct an exam. For the most part, in larger, urban hospitals administrative difficulties in scheduling appointments for crowded clinics often meant that a patient would have to return several times to complete the exam. In contrast, in smaller, rural VA hospitals, driving distances were often so great as practically to require that the exam be done in a single day. Administrative matters such as these were not standardized, and each VA facility was compelled to make its own best local arrangements to accommodate the research study.

That such administrative and other site-to-site differences would contribute to exam variability was recognized from the outset of the study. Because it was impossible to eliminate this variability, the study's strategy was to attempt to limit it (through the directives in the VA circulars) and examine it. For this latter purpose, study staff made site visits to more than 30 VA facilities to explain the research to VA field personnel, answer their questions about the conduct of the study, and gain an appreciation of the actual process by which the examination data were being collected. At each visit, study staff met with the POW physician and administrative coordinators, as well as with other available personnel, and attempted to "walk through" a typical examination. Appendix B contains a list of site visits.

When the study was designed, it was known that a great deal of information would be collected about each participant, given the advancing age of the study groups and especially of the WW II veterans. The volume of data collected was considerable, as Table 4.1 illustrates. The table displays the mean number of diagnoses per examination by study group and indicates, among other things, that examinations of PWK group members each averaged nearly 70 codable medical conditions; the smallest average among the POW groups was nearly 60. Veteran controls averaged markedly fewer

TABLE 4.1 Number of Medical Conditions[a] Among Former POWs of World War II (WW II) and the Korean Conflict and Veteran Controls (mean ± 2 standard errors, *N* in parentheses)

War Era	POWs	Veteran Controls
WW II, Pacific	62.5 ± 4.2 (250)	45.4 ± 6.2 (54)
WW II, Europe	58.4 ± 5.2 (142)	35.2 ± 7.6 (27)
WW II, Europe, malnourished	66.9 ± 6.2 (83)	N.a.
Korean conflict	69.3 ± 3.8 (408)	49.0 ± 5.3 (103)

N.a., not applicable

[a]Number of current and past medical conditions coded from the comprehensive medical examination.

diagnoses than their comparable POWs in every case, but among WP and WK groups, the average number of conditions was still from 45 to nearly 50. Every mention of a medical condition is included in the above counts; if a condition is mentioned in more than one section of the exam (see below), it is counted each time. Such crude data are not meant to represent meaningful differences among study groups. Still, they show the magnitude of information collected and hint at the average "disease burden" of study subjects.

The great volume of data collected, as reflected in the large average number of medical conditions, made it difficult to distinguish the effects of normal aging from the sequelae of military captivity. It was assumed that the critical differentiation of historical and current medical conditions could be made easily, using one part of the examination, the "summary sheet." The sheet was meant to be filled out by the POW physician coordinator as part of an "exit interview" for each examinee; presumably, it would contain all current medical conditions of interest.

Once analysis began, however, it became apparent that about one in seven examinations had no summary section and that the number of medical conditions mentioned on summary sheets constituted only about 15% of the total diagnostic information. This figure was lower than those for the history (21%), findings (24%), and consultation (18%) sections of the exam, but higher than the figures for the sections on psychiatric exams (8%), lab and x-ray (6%), and VA benefits forms (8%). It was not possible, therefore, to derive complete medical data from any one examination section, and some of the analyses in later chapters will be source dependent. For the remainder of this chapter, data on medical conditions were taken from all parts of the exam.

The simplest way to display such data is to categorize them into the customary broad diagnostic categories of the ICD-9-CM classification scheme (e.g., category I, infectious diseases, are all codes from 001 to 139.8; category II, neoplasms, are codes from 140 to 208.9; etc.). For each individual, each coded medical condition is assigned to one of these broad ICD rubrics, but multiple medical conditions within a single category are counted only once, so that the final categorization tells simply the presence or absence of a certain type of medical condition in a person.

The resulting individual data can then be aggregated to calculate *lifetime prevalence rates* (Kleinbaum et al., 1982), although strictly speaking, these might better have been called cumulative lifetime prevalence rates because the lives of these subjects are not yet completed. By the customary definition, a lifetime prevalence rate is the probability that a person has ever had some given medical condition; it is calculated simply by dividing the number of subjects in a group who have ever had that condition by the total number of people in the group.

The examination of the descriptive data in Table 4.2, which contains POW and control lifetime prevalence rates, is hampered by lack of knowledge concerning the stability or, conversely, the variability of these rates. Statistical tests are customarily used to compare such rates because a statistical test takes into account not only the magnitude of differences in rates but also the variability of the rates based on the size of the sample. Given the low response rates (discussed in detail in Chapter 3), however, the customary use of statistical tests would be inappropriate here.

Yet without statistical tests, there is no convenient yardstick with which to determine whether a given difference in prevalence rates is noteworthy. If it is recognized that a statistical test done in this setting has no valid inferential use but is instead merely a way of marking more "noteworthy" or "appreciable" differences, then the usual statistical machinery can be pressed into service in this unusual setting. Thus, statistical tests—specifically the chi-square test—will be used to single out appreciable differences, even though they cannot be labeled "significant."

Additionally on the subject of statistical tests, it should be noted that even the limited use of a statistical test as a marker has the same liability that it has when used in appropriate settings; it customarily classifies differences as either noteworthy or not noteworthy without any gradation between the two. Moreover, a statistical test may conclude that a difference is not noteworthy simply because sample sizes are small (even though the samples are representative); the test is then said to have low power. In the specific case of WW II POW-versus-control comparisons, the very small number of control examinations provides little power to detect and label prevalence rate differences as noteworthy. Finally, in presenting the results of significance tests applied to the data in Table 4.2, it should be remembered that more than 90 such tests were done. By the laws of chance, approximately four "noteworthy" differences would be expected when comparing rates that differed only by random sampling error.

In Table 4.2, the PWP group displays an appreciably higher rate of other endocrine disease (this category includes current and historical nutritional deficiencies) and nervous system disease, as well as an appreciably higher rate of neuroses than the WP group; however, PWP has an appreciably lower rate of blood diseases. PWE and PWEM both display appreciably higher rates of psychoses, neuroses, and injuries or poisonings (almost exclusively injuries), and PWEM an appreciably higher rate of urogenital disease. The PWK group shows the greatest number of noteworthy differences—compared with the WK control group—with elevated rates of infectious disease, other endocrine disease, psychoses, neuroses, nervous system, acute respiratory, digestive, and musculoskeletal disease, as well as injury and poisoning (again, almost exclusively injuries). Like PWP, they show an appreciably lower rate of blood diseases. It should be noted that the

TABLE 4.2 Lifetime Prevalence Rates (percentages) of Medical Conditions Ascertained Through Examination, by ICD Rubric[a] and Study Group

ICD Rubric	PWP	PWE	PWEM	PWK	WP	WE	WK
Infectious diseases	96.4	96.5	98.8	98.0	100.0	92.6	94.2[b]
Malignant neoplasms	20.0	19.7	16.9	9.1	13.0	22.2	12.6
Benign neoplasms	15.6	15.5	19.3	17.7	25.9	14.8	13.6
Diabetes	14.8	13.4	12.1	12.8	18.5	11.1	10.7
Other endocrine diseases	85.6[b]	68.3	81.9	70.8[b]	66.7[b]	70.4	50.5[b]
Blood diseases	14.0[b]	11.3	7.2	12.0[b]	29.6[b]	14.8	22.3[b]
Psychoses	19.6	15.5[b]	24.1[b]	23.0[b]	9.3	0.0[b]	10.7[b]
Neuroses	91.2[b]	88.7[b]	90.4[b]	93.1[b]	79.6[b]	63.0[b]	83.5[b]
Nervous system	36.4[b]	18.3	22.9	25.3[b]	18.5[b]	11.1	11.7[b]
Sense organs	86.8	85.9	86.8	88.2	90.7	77.8	83.5
Heart disease	62.0	60.6	59.0	51.2	66.7	63.0	54.4
Cerebrovascular disease	8.4	9.2	12.1	5.2	1.9	0.0	8.7
Hypertension and other circulatory disease	78.4	71.8	79.5	68.6	66.7	66.7	68.9
Acute respiratory	36.4	26.7	31.3	35.8[b]	25.9	33.3	24.3[b]
Chronic respiratory	68.4	65.5	67.5	61.0	64.8	59.3	56.3
Digestive	94.4	90.1	91.6	94.4[b]	87.0	81.5	83.5[b]
Urogenital	60.4	54.2[b]	49.4	47.1	66.7	33.3[b]	44.7
Skin	75.2	71.1	79.5	70.3	72.2	63.0	66.0
Musculoskeletal	93.6	86.6	89.2	92.4[b]	88.9	81.5	85.4[b]
Congenital conditions	8.0	4.9	7.2	5.6	3.7	3.7	3.9
Symptoms and ill-defined conditions	98.8	97.9	98.8	99.3[b]	98.2	100.0	94.2[b]
Injury and poisoning	85.6	84.5[b]	91.6[b]	91.4	81.5	66.7[b]	94.2
V-codes[c]	52.4	54.9	57.8	50.5	46.3	55.6	54.4
N	250	142	83	408	54	27	103

PWP, prisoner of war, Pacific theater, WW II; PWE, prisoner of war, European theater, WW II; PWEM, prisoner of war, malnourished, European theater, WW II; PWK, prisoner of war, Korean conflict; WP, war veteran, Pacific theater, WW II; WE, war veteran, European theater, WW II; WK, wounded war veteran, Korean conflict.

[a]Coded in ninth revision, International Classification of Disease, Clinical Modification.
[b]Noteworthy (see text) difference between POW and comparable control group.
[c]Factors influencing health status and contact with health services.

PWK and WK groups contain the most examinations, which could well affect the larger number of noteworthy differences (see the discussion of statistical power above). In addition, the PWP group, like the PWK, has somewhat higher, but not noteworthy, rates of digestive disease.

When faced with so many results, one needs to look for consistency across group comparisons and to draw on external results to assess clinical plausibility. For example, the fact that neuroses and psychoses are elevated in nearly all comparisons, coupled with the knowledge that previous studies have shown that psychological illness is found at higher rates among POWs, argues that the apparently increased rates of psychoses and neuroses are more likely to be a real and important clinical difference. In interpreting these apparently very high rates, it should be noted that the psychoses category of ICD-9-CM includes major depression and drug psychoses, such as drug withdrawal syndrome and pathological drug intoxication. The neuroses category includes anxiety states, neurotic depression, depressive disorder, and posttraumatic stress disorder, all later shown individually to be highly prevalent.

Similarly, an elevated rate of other endocrine disease, a category that comprises the nutritional deficiencies, is consistent over several POW groups, as are the elevated rates of injuries among POWs. Other isolated findings, particularly those in the PWK group, are more difficult to interpret, although the somewhat elevated rate of digestive disease in the PWP group and the studies of Australian prisoners of war (which found a higher lifetime rate of ulcer) together argue that this finding has an underlying clinical basis. The most puzzling of the findings common to more than one group is the appreciably lower rate of blood diseases among PWP and PWK. Further discussion of this finding is undertaken in Chapter 6. Given the potential importance of consistency of findings, one can further note that Table 4.2 shows few large differences among disease rates for POWs, despite the somewhat younger age of those in the PWK group compared with the WW II veterans in the PWP and PWE groups. Age differences are not an explicit consideration in the POW-versus-control comparisons because control groups were selected to have the same age distribution as their respective POW samples.

Given the importance of external comparisons, this chapter ends by comparing examination-based lifetime prevalence rates for selected conditions with similar rates from Eberly and Engdahl's (1991) examination study of some 426 former POWs seen at the Minneapolis VA Medical Center. These 426 POWs represented some 60% of the 696 POWs known to be living in the region, and participants in the Minneapolis study were comparable to nonparticipants in terms of age, education, marital status, and military service–connected disability status. The Minneapolis examinations were conducted between April 1984 and April 1987, somewhat early in the course of the MFUA study, which limits the overlap of the Minneapolis and MFUA examination data to only 8 POWs.

Like the lifetime prevalence estimates from the MFUA study, those from the Eberly and Engdahl study are based on a single, comprehensive examination that collected current and historical information. POWs were randomly assigned to one of ten examining psychiatrists, all of whom were experienced in examining and diagnosing psychiatric illnesses in POWs and combat veterans. The psychiatrists collected information on the POW's premilitary history, military and POW experiences, postmilitary adjustment, and current psychiatric status. Historical and current diagnoses were based on this information.

For roughly two-thirds of the 426 Minneapolis exams, the examining psychiatrist used either the Research Diagnostic Criteria of the SADS-L (Spitzer et al., 1978) or a PTSD checklist. The remaining one-third of the sample was reviewed by Eberly and Engdahl, who found that frequencies of the diagnoses obtained using the SADS-L and PTSD checklist were comparable to frequencies later obtained by record review. A sample of 30 cases was rated using both methods, and there was complete agreement between the two in 23 (77%) of these cases. The lifetime prevalence estimates for somatic disorders were derived after experienced coding personnel reviewed the entire medical exam and coded all disorders using the VA's coding system for medical compensation.

Unlike the MFUA study, the Minneapolis study did not include veteran controls. Instead, Eberly and Engdahl compared their findings to lifetime prevalence rates available from a number of studies of selected conditions in the general population (National Institute on Aging, 1986; Weissman and Myers, 1978; Robins et al., 1984; Helzer et al., 1987). For comparison purposes, the following discussion of MFUA examination data will be limited to these same selected medical conditions, and the general population rates cited by Eberly and Engdahl will also be displayed.

Table 4.3 compares lifetime prevalence rates of selected medical and psychiatric conditions for POWs and controls in the MFUA study, POWs in the Minneapolis study, and the general population; the selected conditions shown are those chosen by Eberly and Engdahl. Despite the crude nature of these data (both WW II and Korean conflict POWs are combined, for example), there is a remarkable degree of agreement across all groups. Among the medical conditions, with the exception of intermittent claudication (discussed in detail later in this report), the MFUA data for POWs and controls and the general population data are virtually equivalent. Among Minneapolis POWs, only the lifetime prevalence rate of hypertension is virtually identical to those for MFUA POWs and controls and the general population; for diabetes, cerebrovascular accident, and myocardial infarct, the rates for Minneapolis POWs all seem a bit low in comparison.

Among psychiatric conditions, with the exception of posttraumatic stress disorder (PTSD) and depressive symptoms in MFUA POWs, there is a similar congruence of lifetime prevalence rates (only schizophrenia in MFUA controls appears exceptionally low)—although sample sizes are quite small. It is reasonable to assume that somewhat different diagnostic schemes ac-

TABLE 4.3 Lifetime Prevalence Rates (percentages) of Medical and Psychiatric Diagnoses Among All POWs and Controls in the MFUA Cohort, Among All POWs in the Minneapolis Study, and in the General Population

Diagnosis	MFUA POWs	Minneapolis POWs	MFUA Controls	General Population
Medical conditions				
Hypertension	44.6	39.2	40.2	40.4
Diabetes mellitus	13.4	8.9	13.0	13.2
Cerebrovascular accident	6.2	0.9	5.5	6.4
Myocardial infarction	17.9	7.6	19.6	15.5
Intermittent claudication	13.9	1.9	7.6	2.1
Psychiatric conditions				
Major or minor depression[a]	57.6[a]	23.3	20.7[a]	16.5
Bipolar I or II disorder	0.5	0.9	0.5	1.2
Alcohol abuse or dependence	23.6	21.1	23.4	18.2
Schizophrenia	2.3	1.9	0.5	1.1
Posttraumatic stress disorder	35.9	70.9	9.2	0.5
Number examined	883	426	184	N.a.

N.a, not applicable.

[a]For the MFUA cohort, depression or depressive disorder.

SOURCE: Eberly and Engdahl (1991).

count for most of these differences. For example, the SADS-L criteria used in the Minneapolis study were probably stricter than the simple diagnosis of depressive symptoms used in the MFUA study—certainly the SADS-L criteria were more uniformly applied—and this would explain the lower rate of depression in the Minneapolis cohort. The difference in PTSD rates is more difficult to explain, although the analyses presented in Chapter 5 show that the rates of PTSD vary appreciably by measurement instrument. There is an important comorbidity of PTSD and depressive symptoms, which can also make such comparisons more difficult.

The medical conditions of Table 4.3 are shown in Table 4.4 for all POWs and controls broken down into war period and theater. (This is a reasonable exercise because known differences in age, length of captivity, and harshness of treatment during captivity make it likely that lifetime prevalence rates vary among study groups.) In addition to the conditions listed in Table 4.3, ulcer and general anxiety are included (as they were by Eberly and Engdahl), as well as dysentery, malaria, beriberi, and frozen

TABLE 4.4 Lifetime Prevalence Rates (percentages) of Medical and Psychiatric Diagnoses Among POWs and Controls in the MFUA Cohort and Among POWs in the Minneapolis Study, by Study Group

	MFUA POWs				MFUA Controls			Minneapolis POWs		
Diagnosis	PWP	PWE	PWEM	PWK	WP	WE	WK	PWP	PWE	PWK
Medical conditions										
Hypertension	52.4[a]	42.3	51.8	39.2	37.0	40.7	41.8	42	39	39
Diabetes mellitus	14.8	13.4	12.1	12.8	18.5	11.1	10.7	N.a.	N.a.	N.a.
Cerebrovascular accident	7.6	5.6	9.6	4.9	1.9	0.0	8.7	0	1	0
Myocardial infarction	20.0	19.7	24.1	13.5	24.1	11.1	19.4	19	21	22
Intermittent claudication	17.6	9.2	14.5	13.2	11.1	3.7	6.8	3	2	0
Dysentery	47.2[a]	25.4[a]	37.4[a]	42.9[a]	7.4	3.7	5.8	20	3	11
Malaria	60.8	2.8	1.2	20.6	50.0	7.4	22.3	54	3	11
Beriberi	61.2[a]	0.0	6.2	25.7[a]	0.0	0.0	1.0	48	<1	17
Frozen feet	10.0	16.2	38.6[a]	30.6[a]	1.9	14.8	8.7	5	17	11
Ulcer	19.6	20.4	24.1	26.0[a]	20.4	14.8	15.5	N.a	N.a.	N.a.
Psychiatric conditions										
Depressive disorder[b]	52.4[a]	35.9[a]	53.0[a]	56.4[a]	16.7	0.0	28.2	31	22	28
Bipolar I or II disorder	0.8	0.0	0.0	0.5	1.9	0.0	0.0	3	<1	0
Alcohol abuse or dependence	19.6	18.3	21.7	28.2	14.8	7.4	32.0	22	22	11
Schizophrenia	1.2	0.7	2.4	3.4	0.0	0.0	1.0	3	2	6
Posttraumatic stress disorder	40.8[a]	23.2	27.7	39.0[a]	3.7	11.1	11.7	79	70	53
Generalized anxiety	44.0[a]	46.5[a]	62.7[a]	58.6[a]	13.0	7.4	25.2	58	47	44
Number examined	250	142	83	54	27	103	408	65	343	18

PWP, prisoner of war, Pacific theater, WW II; PWE, prisoner of war, European theater, WW II; PWEM, prisoner of war, malnourished, European theater, WW II; PWK, prisoner of war, Korean conflict; WP, war veteran, Pacific theater, WW II; WE, war veteran, European theater, WW II; WK, wounded war veteran, Korean conflict.

N.a., not applicable.

[a]Noteworthy (see text) difference between POWs and comparable control group.
[b]For Minneapolis POWs, major or minor depression.

feet, conditions that are all known to be linked to harshness of treatment during captivity.

Table 4.4 shows only two medical conditions not associated with prison camp treatment that have appreciably higher prevalences among POWs than controls in the MFUA study: hypertension (in the PWP group) and ulcer (in the PWK). Dysentery is the only prison camp symptom appreciably elevated in all four MFUA POW groups, with beriberi and frozen feet markedly elevated in two of the four groups; there were no noteworthy differences between POWs and controls for lifetime malaria prevalence. The prevalence of cerebrovascular accident appears high in the WK group, especially compared with WP and WE, but it is based on a small sample and is therefore not appreciably higher than the PWK rate (or the PWP, PWE, or PWEM rates). Given the general agreement among all the latter rates, it may be that WP and WE cerebrovascular prevalence rates are unusually low—these are both based on very small samples—rather than the WK rates being unusually high.

Psychiatric conditions are a different matter, with depressive disorder and generalized anxiety showing appreciably higher prevalence rates across all four MFUA POW groups; the rate of 0% among WE is probably attributable to small ($N = 27$) sample size. PTSD is markedly elevated in PWP and PWK and is somewhat higher, although not appreciably so, in PWEM. None of the other psychiatric disorders showed an appreciably higher lifetime prevalence among POWs. Chapters 5 and 6 present a more detailed analysis of the examination data, as well as of the structured psychiatric interview and psychological data. Further discussion of the Eberly and Engdahl data can be found in Chapter 7.

REFERENCES

Eberly RE, Engdahl BE. 1991. Prevalence of somatic and psychiatric disorders among former prisoners of war. Hosp. Commun. Psychiatry 42:807-813.

Helzer JE, Robins LN, McEvoy L. 1987. Post-traumatic stress disorder in the general population. N. Engl. J. Med. 317:1630-1634.

Kleinbaum DG, Kupper LL, Morgenstern H. 1982. Epidemiologic Research: Principles and Quantitative Methods, Van Nostrand Reinhold, New York, p. 118.

National Institute on Aging. 1986. Established Populations for Epidemiological Studies of the Elderly. NIH publication 86-2443. Washington, D.C., U.S. Government Printing Office.

Robins LN, Helzer JE, Weissman MM, et al. 1984. Lifetime prevalence of specific psychiatric disorders at three sites. Arch. Gen. Psychiatry 41:949-958.

Spitzer RL, Endicott J, Robin E. 1978. Research Diagnostic Criteria: rationale and reliability. Arch. Gen. Psychiatry 35:773-782.

Weissman MM, Myers JK. 1978. Affective disorders in a U.S. urban community: the use of the Research Diagnostic Criteria in an epidemiologic survey. Arch. Gen. Psychiatry 35:1304-1311.

5

Examination of Basic Research Questions

Before this research study was begun, five basic research questions (A–E) were formulated as a priori areas of interest. These questions were developed at the time that the 1984–1985 questionnaire follow-up was being completed and were thus heavily influenced by its preliminary results. In brief, those results showed that depressive symptoms were elevated among former POWs, and this finding, along with similar results from Beebe's earlier follow-up (1975), highlighted the need to focus attention first and foremost on psychiatric morbidity. The 1984–1985 results, however, could not provide any real evidence regarding underlying diagnoses—for example, whether the elevated depressive symptoms were associated with a diagnosis of major depression or with, perhaps, posttraumatic stress disorder (PTSD). The hypothesis that PTSD was a probable candidate for either an underlying diagnosis or comorbid condition led eventually to the inclusion of additional psychological questionnaires in the current examination study. Thus, question A focused the study's primary attention on psychiatric morbidity, noting the different methods—physician interview and psychological evaluation—by which these data would be collected. The obvious concern with possible differences in findings based on data collected using the two methods led naturally to question B.

In contrast to psychiatric morbidity, at the time the study was designed there was, by and large, little current information on physical morbidity. Studies of Australian POWs under the Japanese, for example, discovered only one statistically significant difference—an increased history of ulcer—

between those POWs and a comparable group of WW II veteran controls (Goulston et al., 1985); psychiatric findings were much more prominent (Tennant et al., 1986; Dent et al., 1987). Beebe's earlier (1975) study, however, identified a number of conditions with significantly higher hospitalization rates among POWs; more generally, he also found that PWP illness rates were slightly higher than PWK rates and much higher than PWE rates. Thus, question C focused broadly on levels of illness, generally specified, and the main thrust of the question was directed toward determining whether Beebe's earlier findings (1975) on illness differentials still held.

Question D was in the broadest sense a holdover from the 1984–1985 follow-up. At the time of the follow-up, there were nagging questions about the quality of the self-reported data on illnesses, and it was decided that their analysis should be postponed until the more solid examination data were available for comparison. Thus, question D was formulated to emphasize the comparison of self-reported and examination data, and the data presented on question D generally support the original reluctance to analyze the self-reported data alone.

Question E, like others already discussed, was framed with findings from the 1984–1985 follow-up in mind, which had shown that malnourished WW II prisoners of the European theater had significantly elevated depressive symptoms compared with other European prisoners. The malnourished group, however, had not been included in Beebe's 1967 follow-up; consequently, less was known about their physical health in detail. Question E was thus formulated to study broadly the physical health of malnourished PWE.

Before turning to each of the above questions, some discussion of statistical testing is necessary. As was the case in Chapter 4, a useful examination of the descriptive data on POW and control lifetime prevalence rates requires some knowledge of the stability or, conversely, variability of these rates. Statistical tests are customarily used to compare such rates because a statistical test takes into account not only the magnitude of differences in rates but also the variability of the rates based on the size of the sample. Given the low response rates (see Chapter 3), however, the customary use of statistical tests would be inappropriate here. As in Chapter 4, statistical tests will nonetheless be used as indicators of whether a given difference in prevalence rates is "noteworthy" or "appreciable." In doing this, it is recognized that a statistical test done in this setting has no valid inferential use but is instead merely a way of marking such noteworthy or appreciable differences. The additional comments made in Chapter 4 on the limitations of these tests all apply here as well; that is, the tests only mark a difference as noteworthy or not, without gradation; they may conclude that a difference is "not noteworthy" simply because sample sizes are small ("low power"); when a large number of such tests are done, the probability increases that some differences will be wrongly designated as noteworthy by chance.

The sections that follow examine each of the original five questions in turn.

QUESTION A

Will rates of psychiatric illness, as ascertained by interview and psychological evaluation, be higher among former WW II PWP (prisoners of war, Pacific) than among their nonprisoner controls? Will this also hold true for WW II PWE (prisoners of war, European) and PWK (prisoners of war, Korean conflict) when compared with their respective controls? Will rates of psychiatric illness be higher among PWP and PWK than among PWE, as observed in earlier studies?

Based on previous studies of this cohort, it was expected that psychiatric sequelae would continue to persist. The preliminary findings in Chapter 4 clearly support that expectation: all POW groups had appreciably higher lifetime prevalence rates of depression and PTSD, and there is even the suggestion that schizophrenia might be found at a higher rate among POWs than among corresponding controls. In addition to these examination data, however, there are other data on psychiatric sequelae.

The 1984–1985 follow-up found that depressive symptoms were significantly elevated among former POWs, and a hypothesis was formed that these elevated symptoms might be due to or associated with a higher prevalence of PTSD in former POWs. Therefore, this section begins with an examination of the supplemental data on PTSD (see Chapter 2 for details), starting with the PTSD portion of the SCID (*s*tructured *c*linical *i*nterview for *D*SM-III-R); it then moves to one of the four self-administered psychological questionnaires, the Mississippi PTSD scale.

The SCID was designed to be administered by a VA psychiatrist or psychologist, and instructions for its administration directed that it was "to be embedded into the usual POW protocol psychiatric consultation, which should be conducted in the psychiatrist's own practiced manner and style." During data validation checks for this report, however, it was discovered that some of the SCID forms had apparently been given directly to subjects and completed by them. This discovery led to the checking of all completed SCID forms and the removal of those that were apparently self-administered (these amounted to roughly 7% of the total). Data from the remaining SCIDs, presumably administered during the psychiatric interview, are shown in Table 5.A.1.

The SCID measures both current and lifetime rates of PTSD; both are displayed in the table. Although the data show higher lifetime rates of PTSD for PWP, PWE, PWEM, and PWK compared with their respective

TABLE 5.A.1 Lifetime and Current Prevalence Rates (percentages) of Posttraumatic Stress Disorder as Measured by SCID[a], by Study Group

	Lifetime Prevalence (*N*)		Current Prevalence (*N*)	
War Era	POWs	Controls	POWs	Controls
WW II, Pacific	33.3[b] (54)	8.8 (34)	17.3[b] (52)	3.0 (33)
WW II, Europe	23.3 (43)	13.3 (15)	11.6 (43)	13.3 (15)
WW II, Europe, malnourished	31.3 (16)	N.a.	18.8 (16)	N.a.
Korean conflict	41.3 (104)	32.7 (55)	37.9[b] (103)	17.0 (53)

N.a., not applicable.

[a]SCID, Structured Clinical Interview for DSM-III-R.
[b]Appreciable difference in POW and control prevalence.

controls, only the PWP difference is noteworthy. Similarly, there are higher rates of current PTSD for all POW groups (comparing PWEM to WE) but appreciable differences only for PWP and PWK. Overall, the lifetime rates are approximately the same as those found during examination (see Chapter 4), but they are notably lower than those shown for Eberly and Engdahl's study (again, in Chapter 4). Also, in general, lifetime rates of PTSD are all quite higher than current rates, except for the PWK and WE groups. The apparently high rate of current PTSD among WE is somewhat unexpected and may be due to the quite small sample size on which the estimate is based. A more detailed comparison of psychological and interview results is discussed in the section on Question B, later in this chapter.

Another measurement of (current) PTSD, the Mississippi PTSD scale, was also administered as part of the examination, and Table 5.A.2 displays the prevalence rates of current PTSD based on data from that scale. In contrast to Table 5.A.1, rates are appreciably higher for all POW groups, relative to their corresponding controls. It is noteworthy that the rates in Table 5.A.2 are somewhat higher than those for current PTSD ascertained by the SCID; again, this discrepancy will be analyzed in more detail in the discussion of Question B.

The preliminary data in Chapter 4 highlighted depressive symptoms as another psychological condition found at an apparently higher rate among former POWs. Table 5.A.3 displays data on depressive symptoms as ascertained by two independent psychological instruments, the Beck and Center for Epidemiologic Studies depression (CES-D) scales. The Beck scale is designed to characterize depressive symptoms as mild, moderate, or high; however, the data in Table 5.A.3 tabulate the presence only of moderate and high levels of symptoms. These data show that PWP, PWEM, and PWK all have appreciably higher rates of high or moderate depressive symptoms than their respective controls (both PWE and PWEM are compared with PWE); the PWE rate is elevated, but not appreciably so.

As noted earlier, the CES-D scale was administered by mail in the 1984–1985 survey whose results showed depressive symptom prevalence rates roughly three to five times higher among POWs than in other studies of comparable populations. The data in Table 5.A.3 are in line with those of the earlier survey, showing apparently similar rates of depressive symptoms, and all POW groups show appreciably higher levels of depressive symptoms than their respective controls. The WK control group apparently has a much higher rate of depressive symptoms than the WE control group and a slightly higher rate than the WP group; as noted earlier, this may be because this control group consists of combat veterans who were wounded and returned to action.

Table 5.A.4 displays data for the 90-item Hopkins Symptom Check List (SCL-90), scored in the customary manner to yield nine symptom scores plus an "additional items" score, a global severity index (basically, the sum of the individual symptom scores), and a positive symptom distress index (the total score divided by the number of positive items). Comparing PWP, PWEM, and PWK with their control groups, one sees appreciably higher scores for all symptom indices (except the positive symptom index in PWP). Comparing PWE with WE, one sees elevations in scores for somatization, depression, anxiety, interpersonal sensitivity, hostility, and global symptom index.

Looking across POW groups, the PWK group generally has the highest level for every score, with most of their scores strikingly higher than all the others. Next are the PWEM scores, followed closely by PWP scores, with

TABLE 5.A.2 Current Prevalence Rates (percentages) of Posttraumatic Stress Disorder (PTSD) as Measured by the Mississippi PTSD Scale Questionnaire, by Study Group

War Era	POWs	Veteran Controls
WW II, Pacific	32.3[a] (164)[b]	9.3 (86)
WW II, Europe	21.6[a] (111)	5.4 (37)
WW II, Europe, malnourished	38.2[a] (55)	N.a.
Korean conflict	45.4[a] (258)	22.4 (179)

N.a., not applicable.

[a]Appreciable difference in POW and control prevalence.
[b]*N*s appear in parentheses.

TABLE 5.A.3 Depressive Symptoms Among Former POWs and Controls (percentages)

	Beck Score[a] (*N*)		CES-D Score[b] (*N*)	
War Era	POWs	Controls	POWs	Controls
WW II, Pacific	20.3[c] (172)	9.5 (95)	40.1[c] (167)	21.8 (87)
WW II, Europe	15.8 (120)	5.0 (40)	33.3[c] (117)	10.0 (40)
WW II, Europe, malnourished	21.7 (60)	N.a.	47.3[c] (55)	N.a.
Korean conflict	32.5[c] (268)	16.2 (185)	54.1[c] (259)	29.9 (174)

N.a., not applicable.

[a]Beck depression score indicates "high" or "moderate" levels of depressive symptoms.
[b]CES-D, Center for Epidemiologic Studies depression scale. Figures indicate percentage of individuals with a score of 16 or above.
[c]Appreciable difference in POW and control prevalence.

TABLE 5.A.4 Psychological Symptoms Among Former POWs and Controls as Measured by the Hopkins Symptom Checklist (SCL-90) (mean scores)

Symptom	PWP *N*=172	WP *N*=95	PWE *N*=120	PWEM *N*=60	WE *N*=40	PWK *N*=264	WK *N*=185
Somatization	1.148[a]	0.839	1.000[a]	1.254[a]	0.446	1.402[a]	1.031
Depression	1.048[a]	0.634	0.868[a]	1.128[a]	0.431	1.314[a]	0.820
Phobia	0.468[a]	0.195	0.309	0.503[a]	0.141	0.705[a]	0.375
Obsession	1.308[a]	0.810	1.054	1.324[a]	0.704	1.479[a]	0.971
Anxiety	0.889[a]	0.434	0.706[a]	0.940[a]	0.325	1.195[a]	0.726
Paranoia	0.863[a]	0.489	0.663	0.900[a]	0.379	1.197[a]	0.772
Interpersonal sensitivity	0.852[a]	0.468	0.665[a]	0.919[a]	0.285	1.188[a]	0.676
Hostility	0.740[a]	0.444	0.602[a]	0.870[a]	0.248	1.168[a]	0.715
Psychoticism	0.611[a]	0.331	0.453	0.643[a]	0.253	0.846[a]	0.490
More items	1.084[a]	0.744	0.903[a]	1.239[a]	0.548	1.350[a]	0.900
Global symptom index	9.049[a]	5.385	7.209[a]	9.723[a]	3.757	11.863[a]	7.444
Positive symptom distress index	0.190	0.169	0.167	0.192[a]	0.152	0.213[a]	0.185

PWP, prisoner of war, Pacific theater, WW II; PWE, prisoner of war, European theater, WW II; PWEM, prisoner of war, malnourished, European theater, WW II; PWK, prisoner of war, Korean conflict; WP, war veteran, Pacific theater, WW II; WE, war veteran, European theater, WW II; WK, wounded war veteran, Korean conflict.

[a]Appreciable difference between POW and control group scores.

PWE and WK scores fairly close together, trailing somewhat the PWEM and PWP scores. WP and WE scores follow, with WP levels a good deal above those of WE. In brief, looking across all the SCL-90 data, POWs show appreciably higher symptom scores than their respective controls, except for four PWE scores. In addition, PWK and PWEM are notable for their generally raised levels of psychological symptoms across all the subscales.

In summary, question A must be answered in the affirmative: psychiatric morbidity, whether assessed by examination, structured interview, or psychological questionnaire, is apparently higher in former POWs than in their respective controls. Particularly striking are the apparently high rates of PTSD and depressive symptoms. Psychiatric morbidity is appreciably higher in WW II prisoners of the Pacific theater and those of the Korean conflict compared with former WW II POWs of the European theater, as observed in earlier follow-ups of these same groups.

QUESTION B

What differences, if any, will there be between psychiatric morbidity assessed by interviewer versus questionnaire? If there are differences, how will they influence the interpretation of results from question A?

As for question A, this section begins with an examination of the data on PTSD. Table 5.B.1 exhibits the comparative data on PTSD from the medical examination and from the SCID structured interview, limiting this comparison to those who had data for both. In the aggregate, the two give roughly equivalent rates of PTSD prevalence—25.9% for the medical exam and 30.7% for the SCID—but it is imperative to compare the two measures on a person-by-person basis. In Table 5.B.1, each subject is categorized into one of four columns based on his *paired* response to the two methods of measuring PTSD. Thus, each individual is either positive/positive by both measures, positive by exam and negative by SCID, positive by SCID and negative by exam, or negative by both. The resulting categorization results in what is called matched pair data, in which each subject provides his own matched responses for the pair of ratings. The matched pair data of Table 5.B.1 show that there are 21 cases in which the examination diagnosed PTSD and the SCID did not, versus 36 in the opposite direction; the matched pair chi-square (McNemar) test denotes this difference as noteworthy.

Looking more closely, however, one notes that almost all of this difference is concentrated among the controls, specifically, the WK controls; for POWs, the exam and SCID data are nearly identical. There are, of course, two competing interpretations for this difference. If the exam is taken as the standard measurement against which the SCID is compared, then the

TABLE 5.B.1 Comparison of PTSD Lifetime Prevalence Measured by Medical Examination Versus SCID, by Study Group

Study Group (*N*)	Exam Pos./ SCID Pos.	Exam Pos./ SCID Neg.	Exam Neg./ SCID Pos.	Exam Neg./ SCID Neg.
PWP (52)	8	9	9	26
PWE (43)	8	1	2	32
PWEM (15)	4	0	1	10
PWK (102)	31	9	10	52
WP (34)	0	1	3	30
WE (14)	1	0	1	12
WK (53)	8	1	10	34
All subjects (313)	60	21	36	196
All POWs (212)	51	19	22	120[a]
Controls (101)	9	2	14	76[b]

PWP, prisoner of war, Pacific theater, WW II; PWE, prisoner of war, European theater, WW II; PWEM, prisoner of war, malnourished, European theater, WW II; PWK, prisoner of war, Korean conflict; WP, war veteran, Pacific theater, WW II; WE, war veteran, European theater, WW II; WK, wounded war veteran, Korean conflict; PTSD, posttraumatic stress disorder; SCID, Structured Clinical Interview for DSM-III-R.

[a]Not a noteworthy (see text) difference.
[b]A noteworthy (see text) difference.

SCID estimates are too high in WK; alternatively, if one considers the SCID the standard measure, this says that the physician examiners may have had a bias against diagnosing PTSD in WK. Based on the data in hand, either interpretation is defensible.

Moving from lifetime to current PTSD, Table 5.B.2 shows a similar comparison between the examination and the SCID. To estimate the prevalence of current PTSD from exam data, however, it is first necessary to exclude past, inactive cases of PTSD. This was done by making use of some additional data collected for each medical condition, namely, a judgment by the nosologist as to whether that condition had been resolved. For purposes of the following analysis, current PTSD was determined by eliminating PTSD diagnoses for which no resolution could be coded as well as those that had been resolved. Only those unresolved PTSD cases, arguably current cases, are included in the examination data tabulated in Table 5.B.2.

In contrast to the comparison of lifetime data, there are no noteworthy differences, for either POWs or controls, between the estimates of current PTSD based on the SCID and on examination. Also in contrast to the lifetime estimates, the overall estimates of current PTSD from the SCID data are slightly lower than the physician-based estimates: 22.1% for all subjects using the SCID and 24.1% using the exam data. Thus, while there was a noteworthy difference between the SCID and medical exam estimates for *lifetime* PTSD—due solely to the WK group, in which SCID estimates were higher—there are no appreciable differences between SCID and exam estimates for *current* PTSD.

Table 5.B.3 shows a similar comparison of examination estimates of PTSD (again, unresolved cases only) and estimates of PTSD using the Mississippi scale. In contrast to the SCID data on current PTSD (Table 5.B.2), overall Mississippi scale estimates of current PTSD are appreciably higher than the examination estimates: 26.4% prevalence by examination versus 32.4% by the Mississippi scale. Comparison of the matched pair data, however, shows no noteworthy difference between the two estimates for POWs; it does show a noteworthy difference between exam and Mississippi estimates for controls.

The final comparison, the SCID data versus the Mississippi scale data, is shown in Table 5.B.4. Overall, the SCID estimate of current PTSD is appreciably lower than the Mississippi scale estimate: 20.6% for the SCID and 27.2% for the Mississippi scale. Comparison of the matched pair data shows an appreciable difference for POWs only, and nearly all of this dif-

TABLE 5.B.2 Comparison of Current PTSD Prevalence Measured by Medical Examination Versus SCID, by Study Group

Study Group (*N*)	Exam Pos./ SCID Pos.	Exam Pos./ SCID Neg.	Exam Neg./ SCID Pos.	Exam Neg./ SCID Neg.
PWP (50)	7	9	2	32
PWE (43)	4	3	1	35
PWEM (15)	2	2	1	10
PWK (101)	28	10	11	52
WP (33)	0	0	1	32
WE (14)	1	0	1	12
WK (51)	5	3	4	39
All subjects (307)	47	27	21	212
All POWs (209)	41	24	15	129[a]
Controls (98)	6	3	6	83[a]

PWP, prisoner of war, Pacific theater, WW II; PWE, prisoner of war, European theater, WW II; PWEM, prisoner of war, malnourished, European theater, WW II; PWK, prisoner of war, Korean conflict; WP, war veteran, Pacific theater, WW II; WE, war veteran, European theater, WW II; WK, wounded war veteran, Korean conflict; PTSD, posttraumatic stress disorder; SCID, Structured Clinical Interview for DSM-III-R. Current examination data are limited to unresolved conditions.

[a]Not a noteworthy (see text) difference.

TABLE 5.B.3 Comparison of Current PTSD Prevalence Measured by Medical Examination Versus Mississippi Scale, by Study Group

Study Group (*N*)	Exam Pos./ Miss. Pos.	Exam Pos./ Miss. Neg.	Exam Neg./ Miss. Pos.	Exam Neg./ Miss. Neg.
PWP (109)	25	17	13	54
PWE (71)	5	8	11	47
PWEM (34)	7	1	6	20
PWK (199)	46	29	46	78
WP (40)	0	0	2	38
WE (18)	0	0	0	18
WK (78)	4	3	13	58
All subjects (549)	87	58	91	313[b]
All POWs (413)	83	55	76	199[a]
Controls (136)	4	3	15	114[b]

PWP, prisoner of war, Pacific theater, WW II; PWE, prisoner of war, European theater, WW II; PWEM, prisoner of war, malnourished, European theater, WW II; PWK, prisoner of war, Korean conflict; WP, war veteran, Pacific theater, WW II; WE, war veteran, European theater, WW II; WK, wounded war veteran, Korean conflict; PTSD, posttraumatic stress disorder. Current examination data are limited to unresolved conditions.

[a]Not a noteworthy (see text) difference.
[b]A noteworthy (see text) difference.

ference is concentrated in the WW II groups. Although the POW and control SCID-versus-Mississippi comparisons give different results from the exam-versus-Mississippi comparisons, in both cases the overall Mississippi estimates are appreciably higher.

Given the relatively good agreement of estimates of lifetime and current PTSD derived from examination and SCID data (except for WK), but the less favorable agreement of estimates of current PTSD for the exam and SCID versus the Mississippi scale, can any firm conclusions be drawn? There are, unhappily, too many problems with nonresponse bias and measurement issues to permit sound conclusions. Nevertheless, it can be stated that the Mississippi estimates are somewhat higher than the exam and SCID estimates, and that appreciable differences, when they occur, seem concentrated in specific war eras: Mississippi estimates are higher than exam estimates in PWK and WK and higher than SCID estimates in WW II POWs. More research is clearly warranted, especially because the Mississippi scale was developed in groups of Vietnam-era veterans and its items may not properly capture PTSD symptoms in older veterans of earlier wars. There may also be a need simply to redefine scale cut-points and to recalibrate this instrument in older veteran populations.

Analyses parallel to those for PTSD were also conducted for depressive symptoms. Here, the psychological tests were the Beck and the CES-D scales, and the comparison examination data were unresolved diagnoses of depressive disorder, including major and minor depression. The data for the Beck scale, shown in Table 5.B.5, are scored in such a way as to characterize depression as none, mild, moderate, or high; for this analysis, only moderate and high levels (combined) are shown. Overall, the examination estimate of depressive disorder was 28.2% versus 22.6% for the Beck scale, and the matched pair data show a noteworthy difference in the two measures only among POWs (33% for the exam versus 26% for the Beck scale). There were no noteworthy matched pair differences for controls.

Table 5.B.6 displays similar data for the CES-D, using the customary cut-off point whereby scores 16 and above are considered positive for depression. Here, in contrast to the Beck scale data, there are large differences in overall prevalence rates (27.7% using exam data and 39.7% using CES-D data) and noteworthy matched pair differences between the two measures for POWs and controls. In all, the CES-D agrees much less closely with the medical exam than does the Beck scale.

TABLE 5.B.4 Comparison of Current PTSD Prevalence Measured by SCID Versus Mississippi Scale, by Study Group

Study Group (*N*)	SCID Pos./ Miss. Pos.	SCID Pos./ Miss. Neg.	SCID Neg./ Miss. Pos.	SCID Neg./ Miss. Neg.
PWP (40)	6	0	9	25
PWE (33)	4	0	4	25
PWEM (13)	2	0	3	8
PWK (92)	21	12	10	49
WP (28)	0	1	2	25
WE (11)	0	1	0	10
WK (40)	4	2	5	29
All subjects (257)	37	16	33	171[b]
All POWs (178)	33	12	26	107[b]
Controls (79)	4	4	7	64[a]

PWP, prisoner of war, Pacific theater, WW II; PWE, prisoner of war, European theater, WW II; PWEM, prisoner of war, malnourished, European theater, WW II; PWK, prisoner of war, Korean conflict; WP, war veteran, Pacific theater, WW II; WE, war veteran, European theater, WW II; WK, wounded war veteran, Korean conflict; PTSD, posttraumatic stress disorder; SCID, Structured Clinical Interview for DSM III R. Current examination data are limited to unresolved conditions.

[a]Not a noteworthy (see text) difference.
[b]A noteworthy (see text) difference.

In summary, the answer to question B is that examination and psychological questionnaire estimates of the prevalence of psychiatric disorders do differ somewhat and in complicated ways. Taking PTSD first, there was fairly good agreement for lifetime and current PTSD estimates between the exam and the SCID, except for the WK group. The overall Mississippi scale estimates of current PTSD were a bit higher than the SCID or exam rates, but such differences appeared to be dependent on war era.

Turning to depression, the CES-D data yield appreciably higher estimates of the prevalence of depressive disorder—more for POWs than for controls—compared with examination data. This may merely reflect the fact that the CES-D was designed to measure depressive symptoms rather than provide a diagnosis of depression. In contrast, the Beck scale data show appreciably lower estimates of the prevalence of depressive disorders for POWs but not controls, compared with the exam data. The exclusion of the "mild" category cases from the analysis may have affected this comparison. Overall, the Beck scale results parallel the physicians' examination diagnoses of depression more closely than do the CES-D scale results.

Notwithstanding the above discussion, POWs show appreciably more

TABLE 5.B.5 Comparison of Prevalence of Current Depression Measured by Medical Examination Versus Beck Scale

Study Group (*N*)	Exam Pos./ Beck Pos.	Exam Pos./ Beck Neg.	Exam Neg./ Beck Pos.	Exam Neg./ Beck Neg.
PWP (117)	9	22	15	71
PWE (47)	8	12	6	54
PWEM (38)	7	7	3	21
PWK (209)	41	42	28	98
WP (43)	0	4	2	37
WE (18)	0	0	0	18
WK (83)	5	9	9	60
All subjects (588)	70	96	63	359[b]
All POWs (444)	65	83	52	244[b]
Controls (144)	5	13	11	115[a]

PWP, prisoner of war, Pacific theater, WW II; PWE, prisoner of war, European theater, WW II; PWEM, prisoner of war, malnourished, European theater, WW II; PWK, prisoner of war, Korean conflict; WP, war veteran, Pacific theater, WW II; WE, war veteran, European theater, WW II; WK, wounded war veteran, Korean conflict. Current examination data are limited to unresolved conditions. Beck depression score indicates "high" or "moderate" levels of depressive symptoms.

[a]Not a noteworthy (see text) difference.
[b]A noteworthy (see text) difference.

TABLE 5.B.6 Comparison of Prevalence of Current Depression Measured by Medical Examination Versus CES-D Scale

Study Group (*N*)	Exam Pos./ CES-D Pos.	Exam Pos./ CES-D Neg.	Exam Neg./ CES-D Pos.	Exam Neg./ CES-D Neg.
PWP (115)	19	11	27	58
PWE (79)	13	7	16	43
PWEM (37)	11	3	7	16
PWK (201)	61	18	46	76
WP (40)	1	2	3	34
WE (20)	0	0	2	18
WK (82)	7	6	16	53
All subjects (574)	112	47	117	298[a]
All POWs (432)	104	39	96	193[a]
Controls (142)	8	8	21	105[a]

PWP, prisoner of war, Pacific theater, WW II; PWE, prisoner of war, European theater, WW II; PWEM, prisoner of war, malnourished, European theater, WW II; PWK, prisoner of war, Korean conflict; WP, war veteran, Pacific theater, WW II; WE, war veteran, European theater, WW II; WK, wounded war veteran, Korean conflict; CES-D, Center for Epidemiologic Studies depression scale. Current examination data are limited to unresolved conditions.

[a]A noteworthy (see text) difference.

psychological problems than their respective controls by all measures. The differences among the various measurements, while of methodological interest and of potential importance when making comparisons with other studies, do not in any material way influence the conclusions drawn earlier in question A.

QUESTION C

How have differences in illness levels changed over time? In particular, have the earlier differentials between the PWP and PWK groups, on the one hand, and the PWP and PWE groups, on the other, decreased with time?

In Beebe's earlier (1975) follow-up, illness levels were higher among PWP than among PWK, in line with repatriation examination data suggesting that PWP sustained greater impairment to their health during captivity than did PWK. On the other hand, PWP illness levels were notably higher than those for PWE, among whom only psychiatric sequelae were apparent. The passage of an additional two decades raises the obvious question: Have these earlier relationships changed?

To answer this question of changes over time requires comparable data from the two time periods. The 1967 follow-up collected data by questionnaire and record review, and such data are not directly comparable to the current medical examination information. However, the 1967 data on hospitalization are fundamentally comparable to similar data collected as part of the 1984–1985 questionnaire follow-up, and it is these data that will be used in the following analysis. Although these hospitalization data provide material for comparison between the two time periods, such data are relatively gross measures of morbidity; for example, many people suffering from mental illness are not hospitalized. Thus, there may be differences between groups that would not be readily apparent in hospital data. In addition, the 1967 data combine self-reported hospitalization data for nonfederal hospitalizations with data from VA and Army files, whereas the 1984–1985 data are strictly self-reported. Also, the earlier data were coded to the seventh revision of the International Classification of Diseases and Injuries, which necessitates the use of broad diagnostic categories when making comparisons with the 1984–1985 data, which were coded to the ninth revision of the International Classification of Diseases, Clinical Modification (ICD-9-CM).

Table 5.C.1 shows the earlier hospitalization data for PWP, PWE, and PWK. (The PWEM group, which was sampled independently of PWE, was not a part of the 1967 follow-up.) Hospital admission rates have been combined for the earlier follow-up periods (1946–1965 for PWP and PWE and 1954–1965 for PWK) to compute an average admission rate, adjusted for length of follow-up, of admissions per 1,000 per year. The data show some quite striking (fivefold or more) differences between PWP and PWE admission rates for infectious disease; allergic, endocrine, and nutritional disorders; and mental diseases; they also show sizable (around twofold) differences in almost every other organ system. Differences between PWP and PWK are on the whole much smaller, with sizable PWP elevations only for allergic and endocrine diseases and mental diseases, and a sizable elevation for PWK in hospitalizations for accidents, injury, and poisonings.

Table 5.C.2 shows later data on hospitalization, during the period 1984–1985, for PWP, PWE, and PWK, plus an additional group, PWEM, again calculated as admissions per 1,000 per year. These data tell a different story. There are no longer any striking differences among the three groups of Table 5.B.1, not even when PWEM is included, and sizable differences persist only for mental disease. PWK hospitalization rates are lower for circulatory disease, a finding that is probably age related, but they are not otherwise uniformly lower than rates for WW II POWs.

Although no definitive interpretation of the data in Tables 5.C.1 and 5.C.2 is possible, three pertinent points should be kept in mind. First, some of the differences seen between PWP and PWK illness levels two decades

TABLE 5.C.1 Rates of Self-Reported Hospitalization from the 1967 Follow-up Study, in Admissions per Thousand Persons per Year, by ICD Rubric[a] and Study Group

ICD Rubric	PWP	PWE	PWK
Infectious diseases	20.1	2.4	15.2
Malignant neoplasms	1.3	0.6	0.3
Benign neoplasms	3.6	3.7	3.3
Allergic and endocrine diseases	11.8	2.1	3.8
Blood diseases	0.6	0.3	0.1
Mental diseases	31.4	7.6	22.1
Nervous system	4.8	0.6	4.2
Sense organs	6.3	1.6	3.8
Circulatory disease	13.8	5.7	11.6
Respiratory	19.2	8.9	21.5
Digestive	25.3	14.9	25.1
Urogenital	8.2	5.5	9.7
Skin	8.7	3.7	10.2
Musculoskeletal	11.8	6.2	7.7
Congenital conditions	0.7	0.0	1.0
Symptoms and ill-defined conditions	16.5	10.9	18.3
Injury and poisoning	19.4	12.7	29.8
Observation and exam[b]	11.6	2.5	9.7

PWP, prisoner of war, Pacific theater, WW II; PWE, prisoner of war, European theater, WW II; PWK, prisoner of war, Korean conflict.

[a]Coded to the seventh revision, International Classification of Diseases.
[b]Comparable to V-codes (i.e., factors influencing health status and contact with health services).

ago could be attributed to age, with the typical PWP being 45–55 years old and the typical PWK 35–45 years old; as both groups age, this chronological difference should become less important. Second, differences in hospital admission rates over time may be due, at least in part, to deaths of the sicker men over time. Third, as one moves further from the time of captivity, one also moves closer to old age, when regardless of earlier health, background levels of illness start to rise dramatically.

Another, less suitable way to look at changes over time is to compare lifetime prevalence rates from the examination with current prevalence rates from the same source, again considering current conditions to be those that are still unresolved. Earlier, Table 4.2 displayed lifetime prevalence rates for all medical conditions in broad ICD rubrics. Table 5.C.3 exhibits cur-

TABLE 5.C.2 Rates of Self-reported Hospitalization from 1984–1985 Follow-up Study, in Admissions per Thousand Persons per Year, by ICD Rubric[a] and Study Group

ICD Rubric	PWP	PWE	PWEM	PWK
Infectious diseases	1.1	0.7	1.3	1.1
Malignant neoplasms	4.6	2.4	1.3	1.2
Benign neoplasms	1.1	0.7	0.3	0.2
Endocrine diseases	1.9	1.7	1.0	1.5
Blood diseases	0.4	0.0	0.3	0.2
Mental diseases	4.5	1.1	4.7	9.2
Nervous system	3.0	2.8	3.4	3.1
Sense organs	2.4	2.0	0.7	1.0
Circulatory disease	26.7	23.6	22.8	18.0
Respiratory	4.5	5.7	4.4	3.7
Digestive	17.5	16.2	18.8	14.3
Urogenital	10.3	7.0	10.1	6.4
Skin	1.4	1.3	1.7	3.0
Musculoskeletal	8.0	8.5	10.4	11.0
Congenital conditions	0.1	0.0	0.0	0.0
Symptoms and ill-defined conditions	4.6	3.0	6.7	7.7
Injury and poisoning	4.5	4.4	2.7	6.7
V-codes[b]	8.3	5.7	7.0	6.4

PWP, prisoner of war, Pacific theater, WW II; PWE, prisoner of war, European theater, WW II; PWEM, prisoner of war, malnourished, European theater, WW II; PWK, prisoner of war, Korean conflict.

[a]Coded to the ninth revision, International Classification of Diseases, Clinical Modification.
[b]Factors influencing health status and contact with health services.

rent prevalence rates in a similar fashion. Categories for which there are noteworthy differences in rates between POWs and controls are so designated.

Table 5.C.3 shows noteworthy differences in the current prevalence of diseases of the blood (the PWP and PWK groups have *lower* levels), other endocrine diseases (the PWP group is *lower*), psychoses (all but PWE), neuroses (all groups), nervous system (PWP and PWK), digestive diseases (PWP and PWK), symptoms (PWK), and V-codes, which are not strictly medical diagnoses but are factors that influence health status and contact with health services (PWP). Because they are ill-defined, the latter two nondisease categories will not be studied further; however, the remaining findings will be reconsidered in Chapter 6. In all, there were 13 noteworthy differences, 5 fewer than seen in Table 4.2; these are summarized in Table 5.C.4. These results support the findings in Tables 5.C.1 and 5.C.2 of lessening health differences over time.

In summary, based on hospitalization data, it appears that differences in illness levels among POW groups have become smaller over time. In the 1967 follow-up, PWP hospitalization rates were somewhat greater than those for PWK and notably larger than those for PWE; by 1984–1985, nearly all readily apparent differences had disappeared. Comparing lifetime and current prevalence data from the exam (a much more indirect measure of change over time) generally supported the hospitalization findings and showed that

TABLE 5.C.3 Prevalence Rates (percentages) of Current Medical Conditions by ICD Rubric[a] and Study Group

ICD Rubric	PWP	PWE	PWEM	PWK	WP	WE	WK
Infectious diseases	22.8	18.3	19.3	27.7	29.6	7.4	20.4
Malignant neoplasms	4.0	2.1	4.8	2.9	1.9	3.7	3.9
Benign neoplasms	11.6	12.0	10.8	10.1	20.4	11.1	9.7
Diabetes mellitus	14.8	13.4	12.1	12.5	18.5	7.4	10.7
Other endocrine diseases	44.8[b]	47.2	50.6	43.1	66.7[b]	70.4	48.5
Blood diseases	12.4[b]	9.9	7.2	11.5[b]	25.9[b]	14.8	21.4[b]
Psychoses	15.2[b]	11.3	18.1[b]	19.1[b]	3.7[b]	0.0[b]	5.8[b]
Neuroses	87.6[b]	82.4[b]	86.8[b]	90.0[b]	74.1[b]	63.0[b]	80.6[b]
Nervous system	31.2[b]	12.0	20.5	21.1[b]	9.3[b]	11.1	7.8[b]
Sense organs	83.6	82.4	84.3	85.1	85.2	74.1	80.6
Heart disease	56.0	56.3	56.6	46.6	57.4	63.0	50.5
Cerebrovascular disease	1.6	1.4	2.4	2.2	0.0	0.0	2.9
Hypertension and other circulatory diseases	75.2	64.1	77.1	63.2	63.0	66.7	61.2
Acute respiratory	4.8	2.8	6.0	2.9	9.3	3.7	2.9
Chronic respiratory	57.6	54.9	57.8	52.7	53.7	44.4	44.7
Digestive	74.4[b]	70.4	74.7	81.6[b]	57.4[b]	70.4	58.3[b]
Urogenital	46.4	35.2	37.4	29.7	44.4	25.9	32.0
Skin	64.8	62.0	73.5	64.2	70.4	63.0	62.1
Musculoskeletal	92.8	84.5	89.2	90.0	85.2	77.8	84.5
Congenital conditions	6.8	4.2	3.6	5.2	3.7	3.7	2.9
Symptoms and ill-defined conditions	97.2	93.7	98.8	98.0[b]	98.2	100.0	92.2[b]
Injury and poisoning	26.4	26.8	21.7	26.7	22.2	18.5	18.5
V-codes[c]	30.8[b]	46.5	42.2	49.3	46.3[b]	55.6	54.4
Number of exams	250	142	83	408	54	27	103

PWP, prisoner of war, Pacific theater, WW II; PWE, prisoner of war, European theater, WW II; PWEM, prisoner of war, malnourished, European theater, WW II; PWK, prisoner of war, Korean conflict; WP, war veteran, Pacific theater, WW II; WE, war veteran, European theater, WW II; WK, wounded war veteran, Korean conflict.

[a]Coded to the ninth revision, International Classification of Diseases, Clinical Modification.
[b]Noteworthy (see text) difference between POW and control prevalence rates.
[c]Factors influencing health status and contact with health services.

TABLE 5.C.4 Study Groups Showing Noteworthy Differences Between POW and Control Prevalence Rates of Lifetime and Current Medical Conditions, by ICD Rubric[a]

ICD Rubric	Lifetime	Current
Infectious diseases	PWK	None
Malignant neoplasms	None	None
Benign neoplasms	None	None
Diabetes mellitus	None	None
Other endocrine diseases	PWP, PWK	PWP
Blood diseases	PWP, PWK	PWP, PWK
Psychoses	PWE, PWEM, PWK	PWP, PWEM, PWK
Neuroses	All groups	All groups
Nervous system	PWP, PWK	PWP, PWK
Sense organs	None	None
Heart disease	None	None
Cerebrovascular disease	None	None
Hypertension and other circulatory diseases	None	None
Acute respiratory	PWK	None
Chronic respiratory	None	None
Digestive	PWK	PWP, PWK
Urogenital	PWE	None
Skin	None	None
Musculoskeletal	PWK	None
Congenital conditions	None	None
Symptoms and ill-defined conditions	PWK	PWK
Injury and poisoning	PWE, PWEM	None
V-codes[b]	None	PWP

PWP, prisoner of war, Pacific theater, WW II; PWE, prisoner of war, European theater, WW II; PWEM, prisoner of war, malnourished, European theater, WW II; PWK, prisoner of war, Korean conflict.

[a]Coded to the ninth revision, International Classification of Diseases, Clinical Modification.
[b]Factors influencing health status and contact with health services.

there were fewer noteworthy current POW-versus-control differences than lifetime differences.

QUESTION D

How do the physician-reported physical examination findings compare with the self-reported diagnoses, symptoms, and complaints from the 1984 questionnaire? Which physical findings are under- or overreported, and how do nonmedical factors influence this reporting?

Although the 1984–1985 questionnaire follow-up was focused on psychiatric morbidity and contained as its centerpiece the Center for Epidemiologic Studies depression scale, it also contained two general items on current health, asking about medical conditions that were and were not being treated. The first item was worded as follows: "Are you currently now under medical care?" It was followed with a "By whom?" Space was then left to list up to five such medical conditions; the subject's responses were coded using ICD-9-CM. The second item asked, "Do you need medical care that you are not receiving?" Again, it was followed by blank spaces for up to five conditions. These data, however, were relatively sparse and are not tabulated here.

Because the levels of reported medical conditions under treatment are roughly comparable across all four POW groups, the data in Table 5.D.1

TABLE 5.D.1 Rates (percentages) of Self-Reported Medical Conditions Treated from the 1984–1985 Questionnaire for All POW Groups, by ICD Rubric[a]

ICD Rubric	Reported Rate
Infectious diseases	2.5
Cancer	4.1
Benign neoplasms	0.4
Diabetes mellitus	4.4
Other endocrine diseases	5.3
Blood diseases	0.4
Psychoses	0.6
Neuroses	9.0
Nervous system	2.7
Sense organs	8.7
Heart disease	15.5
Cerebrovascular disease	1.1
Hypertension and other circulatory diseases	26.9
Acute respiratory	0.3
Chronic respiratory	7.8
Digestive	11.7
Urogenital	4.6
Skin	4.6
Arthritis	13.1
Other musculoskeletal	10.7
Congenital conditions	0.05
Symptoms and ill-defined conditions	23.1
Injury and poisoning	3.1
V-codes[b]	14.9

[a]Coded to the ninth revision, International Classification of Diseases, Clinical Modification.

[b]Factors influencing health status and contact with health services.

show all POW groups combined. To facilitate later comparisons, each of the four POW groups has been given equal weighting. Self-reported rates are, for the most part, under 10% prevalence, with the exceptions of heart disease, hypertension and other circulatory disease, digestive disease, arthritis, other musculoskeletal disease, symptoms and ill-defined conditions, and V-codes.

Before attempting to compare the self-reported data in Table 5.D.1 with examination data, some further discussion is in order. The self-reported data were responses to a question about current medical care, but the examination contains historical as well as current problems. Question B used one potential method of separating current from historical medical exam conditions: selecting only unresolved conditions. In this section, another method in addition to that is used. This second method considers the source of the examination information, coded for every medical condition, and selects information only from certain sources. Because summary diagnosis data, perhaps the single best source of data, were unavailable for many subjects, data from all findings and laboratory sections of the medical examination were combined to produce the exam data. (Both the findings and laboratory sections of the exam were thought to be freer of historical information.) Prevalence rates based on these two combined sources are displayed in Table 5.D.2.

Comparing these two sets of rates, one sees that in general the prevalence rates for unresolved conditions are equal to or greater than the rates for medical conditions in the findings and laboratory sections of the exam. This apparently higher rate is most striking for psychoses, neuroses, and nervous system conditions; only the unresolved acute respiratory conditions have a notably lower rate.

Despite their differences, both the unresolved medical conditions and the medical conditions from the findings and laboratory sections show rates that are strikingly higher than the rates of self-reported medical conditions in Table 5.D.1. To facilitate a rough comparison between self-reported and exam data, *prevalence rate ratios* were calculated by dividing the rates for unresolved and for findings/laboratory medical conditions by the self-reported ones. For ease of calculation and comparison, each of the four POW groups was weighted equally. Both of these ratios are displayed in Table 5.D.3.

Table 5.D.3 shows that, with only two exceptions, every ratio is well above 1, meaning that the examination-based rates are notably higher than the self-reported rates. The ratios, by and large, range between 2 and 10 and are mostly greater for unresolved conditions than for findings/laboratory conditions. Part of the explanation for the lower rates of self-reporting lies in the reporting process itself. First, questionnaire space limited the maximum number of self-reported conditions to five per person, whereas the number of medical examination responses, for both unresolved and findings/laboratory conditions, was essentially unbounded. Although the average number of questionnaire responses was around 3, ranging from 2.9 for PWP to 3.5 for PWE, the critical question—for which data are unavailable—is, how many of those who reported five conditions might have reported six or more? Second, self-reported medical conditions were necessarily reported in less precise layman's language, leading in some cases to artificial differences in rate ratios. For example, V-codes are factors that influence health status; they may include such items as a personal history of

TABLE 5.D.2 Prevalence Rates (percentages) of Medical Conditions Derived from the Findings and Laboratory Sections of the Medical Examination and Statements of Unresolved Medical Conditions, by ICD Rubric[a]

	Prevalence	
ICD Rubric	Findings and Lab Conditions	Unresolved Conditions
Infectious diseases	24.8	22.0
Cancer	9.8	3.5
Benign neoplasms	7.7	11.1
Diabetes mellitus	8.1	13.2
Other endocrine diseases	36.2	46.4
Blood diseases	7.5	10.3
Psychoses	2.5	15.9
Neuroses	48.1	86.7
Nervous system	9.1	21.2
Sense organs	67.6	83.9
Heart disease	43.9	53.9
Cerebrovascular disease	3.9	1.9
Hypertension	48.5	69.9
Acute respiratory	19.6	4.1
Chronic respiratory	44.8	55.8
Digestive	71.2	75.3
Urogenital	32.2	37.2
Skin	44.8	66.1
Arthritis	57.7	74.8
Other musculoskeletal	63.7	78.9
Congenital conditions	2.5	5.0
Symptoms and ill-defined conditions	88.3	96.9
Injury and poisoning	22.9	25.4
V-codes[b]	3.0	42.2
Number of exams	883	883

[a]Coded to the ninth revision, International Classification of Diseases, Clinical Modification.
[b]Factors influencing health status and contact with health services.

TABLE 5.D.3 Prevalence Rate Comparability Ratios for Findings/Laboratory and Unresolved Medical Conditions Versus Self-reported Medical Conditions, by ICD Rubric[a] for all POW Groups Combined

ICD Rubric	Ratio of Findings/Laboratory Medical Conditions to Self-Reported	Ratio of Unresolved Medical Conditions to Self-Reported
Infectious diseases	10.2	8.8
Cancer	2.4	0.8
Benign neoplasms	18.1[b]	26.2[b]
Diabetes mellitus	1.8	3.0
Other endocrine diseases	6.9	8.8
Blood diseases	17.6[b]	24.1[b]
Psychoses	4.3[b]	27.7[b]
Neuroses	5.3	9.6
Nervous system	3.3	7.8
Sense organs	7.8	9.7
Heart disease	2.8	3.5
Cerebrovascular disease	3.5[b]	1.7[b]
Hypertension and other circulatory diseases	1.8	2.6
Acute respiratory	60.2[b]	12.7[b]
Chronic respiratory	5.8	7.2
Digestive	6.1	6.5
Urogenital	7.0	8.1
Skin	9.8	14.5
Arthritis	4.4	5.7
Other musculoskeletal	5.9	7.4
Congenital conditions	[c]	[c]
Symptoms and ill-defined conditions	3.8	4.2
Injury and poisoning	7.4	8.3
V-codes[d]	0.2	2.8

[a]Coded to the ninth revision, International Classification of Diseases, Clinical Modification.
[b]Based on low self-reported rates (under 2.0%).
[c]Self-reported rates were too small to calculate a reliable rate.
[d]Factors influencing health status and contact with health services.

selected conditions (e.g., cancer). When they are self-reported, such medical conditions would be assigned V-codes, but they probably would not be recorded by a physician as an unresolved condition nor included in either the findings or laboratory sections of the examination. It is not surprising, therefore, that V-codes were reported more frequently on a questionnaire than in the findings/laboratory section of the medical examination. Nor is it surprising that self-reporting was most complete (i.e., comparability ratios

TABLE 5.D.4 Rank Ordering of Prevalence Rate Comparability Ratios (in parentheses) for Findings/Laboratory and Unresolved Medical Conditions Versus Self-Reported Medical Conditions, by ICD Rubric[a] for all POW Groups Combined

	Ranking of Ratios of Findings/Laboratory Medical Conditions to Self-Reported	Ranking of Ratios of Unresolved Medical Conditions to Self-Reported
(Highest rates of self-report)	V-codes[b] (0.2)	Cancer (0.8)
	Hypertension and other circulatory diseases (1.8)	Cerebrovascular disease[c] (1.7)
	Diabetes mellitus (1.8)	Hypertension and other circulatory diseases (2.6)
	Cancer (2.4)	V-codes[b] (2.8)
	Heart disease (2.8)	Diabetes mellitus (3.0)
	Nervous system (3.3)	Heart disease (3.5)
	Cerebrovascular disease[c] (3.5)	Symptoms and ill-defined conditions (4.2)
	Symptoms and ill-defined conditions (3.8)	Arthritis (5.7)
	Psychoses[c] (4.3)	Digestive (6.5)
	Arthritis (4.4)	Chronic respiratory (7.2)
	Neuroses (5.3)	Other musculoskeletal (7.4)
	Chronic respiratory (5.8)	Nervous system (7.8)
	Other musculoskeletal (5.9)	Urogenital (8.1)
	Digestive (6.1)	Injury and poisoning (8.3)
	Other endocrine (6.9)	Other endocrine (8.8)
	Urogenital (7.0)	Infectious diseases (8.8)
	Injury and poisoning (7.4)	Neuroses (9.6)
	Sense organs (7.8)	Sense organs (9.7)
	Skin (9.8)	Acute respiratory[c] (12.7)
	Infectious diseases (10.2)	Skin (14.5)
(Lowest rates of self-report)	Blood diseases[c] (17.6)	Blood diseases[c] (24.1)
	Benign neoplasms[c] (18.1)	Benign neoplasms[c] (26.2)
	Acute respiratory[c] (60.2)	Psychoses[c] (27.7)

[a]Coded in ninth revision, International Classification of Diseases, Clinical Modification.
[b]Factors influencing health status and contact with health services.
[c]Based on low self-reported rates (under 2.0%).

were lowest) for chronic conditions that are easily described in less technical language, such as cancer, diabetes, heart disease, and hypertension.

Although comparability ratios tended to be higher for unresolved medical conditions than for medical conditions derived from the findings and laboratory sections of the examination, some of the artifactual problems above make ratio comparisons difficult. To facilitate such comparisons Table 5.D.4 displays the ranking as well as the value of the ratios. The ranked conditions show fairly good agreement between the two columns with the exception of psychoses, for which the ratio of self-reported to findings/laboratory conditions is substantially higher than the ratio of self-reported to unresolved medical conditions; presumably, psychoses are less often resolved. In addition, several of the high-ratio conditions, like psychoses and benign neoplasms, are based on very low self-reported prevalence, which makes their ratios less stable and more prone to error.

In summary, the simple answer to question D is that physician-reported findings appear to be much more frequent than self-reported findings on medical conditions across almost all broad diagnostic categories. Some of that difference can be attributed to the reporting process, in particular, the limitation of five self-reported medical conditions; some differences are accentuated or possibly created by the use of medical versus nonmedical terminology. In more general terms, underreporting may be due to the subjects' lack of understanding of medical conditions or even denial of them. Nonetheless, the differences measured here were sizable and deserve additional future study, along with the question of how nonmedical factors influence differences between physician and self-reported rates.

QUESTION E

Can any distinctive signs of abnormal physical findings be seen in the subset of PWE veterans who were seriously malnourished at repatriation?

The group of WW II European theater POWs designated as PWEM are an independent sample of POWs added by Nefzger (1970) for the second follow-up. The group was derived from a 20% sample of Army hospital admissions with diagnoses of malnutrition; those chosen had no diagnosis other than malnutrition and had remained in the hospital at least 10 days. The comparison of these PWEM to the larger group of all WW II European theater prisoners, PWE, affords an opportunity to study the long-term effects of a relatively short (compared with PWP) period of captivity that nonetheless produced severe malnutrition in its survivors.

The tables pertaining to question A showed that rates of psychological sequelae are clearly higher in PWEM, compared with PWE; the focus of question E, however, is on physical findings. In Chapter 4, lifetime prevalence data for medical conditions were displayed in Table 4.2. These data showed few striking differences between PWEM and PWE, although in general, lifetime prevalence rates across all ICD rubrics were higher for PWEM than for PWE; the only noteworthy difference in PWEM and PWE rates is for "other endocrine disease" (which includes nutritional deficiencies).

Because there were no precise medical hypotheses specified beforehand, the study of broad disease categories in Chapter 4 was defensible as a protection against overlooking unanticipated findings. This high level of diagnostic aggregation also produces larger samples and yields more stable prevalence estimates. Yet such high-level aggregation is not without its problems. In particular, the higher the level of diagnostic aggregation, the greater the likelihood that distinct medical conditions will be put together, thereby increasing the risk of not observing an elevated rate for a narrowly defined condition because it has been combined with other lower rate conditions into a broader category.

One solution to this dilemma, which is discussed again in the next chapter, is to settle on some small, fixed set of narrower diagnostic categories for study. Although there were insufficient data to formulate precise a priori medical hypotheses for question E, a relatively small set of diagnostic categories can be chosen for further study on the basis of recently published POW examination studies. In Chapter 4, the diagnostic categories reported by Eberly and Engdahl (1991) were studied. To these are added other diagnostic categories from the work of Steven Oboler and colleagues of the Denver VA Medical Center, whose findings are based on the examination of some 200 former POWs, mostly veterans of WW II (Oboler, 1987, and subsequent personal communication). Table 5.E.1 shows lifetime prevalence data for the combined Eberly/Engdahl and Oboler categories.

There are five diagnostic categories in which PWEM lifetime prevalence rates appreciably exceed those of PWE. Aside from dysentery, beriberi, and frozen feet—these three are presumably elevated as a result of prison camp medical history—the rates of peripheral nerve disease and gastroenteritis are appreciably elevated. To determine whether some specific diagnoses might account for the above aggregate differences, detailed diagnostic data were examined. Two narrowly defined diagnostic conditions make up the gastroenteritis category: other and unspecified noninfectious gastroenteritis and colitis (ICD-9-CM code 558.9) and irritable colon (ICD-9-CM code 564.1, which includes irritable bowel syndrome). The rates of the latter condition were nearly identical in PWEM and PWE, so that the apparent difference in lifetime prevalence of gastroenteritis is almost all accounted for by a difference in the prevalence of noninfectious gastroenteritis and colitis.

The data for peripheral nerve disease are more complicated. Table 5.E.2 shows the detailed three-digit subcategories and their ICD codes. Although the numbers of cases, and therefore the prevalence rates, are quite low when reported by detailed diagnostic category, it remains clear that most of the excess PWEM peripheral neuropathy is confined to three subcategories. Lifetime prevalence rates of mononeuritis of the upper and lower limbs and hereditary and idiopathic neuropathy together appear to account for most of the PWEM excess. The very sparse numbers of diagnoses here, however, yield rates that must be even more cautiously interpreted than earlier prevalence rates.

TABLE 5.E.1 Number and Lifetime Rate (per hundred) of Selected Diagnoses[a] from the Medical Examination, for PWEM and PWE

	PWEM (N=82)		PWE (N=142)	
Diagnostic Category	Number	Rate	Number	Rate
Hypertension (strictly defined)	43	51.8	60	42.3
Diabetes	10	12.1	19	13.4
Intermittent claudication	12	14.5	13	9.2
Cerebrovascular accident	8	9.6	8	5.6
Dysentery	31	37.4[b]	36	25.4
Malaria	1	1.2	4	2.8
Beriberi	5	6.0[b]	0	0.0
Frozen feet	32	38.6[b]	23	16.2
Ulcer	20	24.1	29	20.4
Myocardial infarct	20	24.1	28	19.7
Asthma	2	2.4	11	7.8
Peripheral nerve disease	15	18.1[b]	12	8.5
Arterial vascular disease	26	31.3	38	26.8
Gastroenteritis	36	43.4[b]	40	28.2
Osteoarthritis	27	32.5	48	33.8
Traumatic arthritis	1	1.2	0	0.0
Chronic obstructive pulmonary disease	12	14.5	22	15.5

PWEM, prisoner of war, malnourished, European theater, WW II; PWE, prisoner of war, European theater, WW II.

[a]Coded to the ninth revision, International Classification of Diseases, Clinical Modification.
[b]Noteworthy (see text) difference between POW and control prevalence rates.

In summary, the answer to question E must be that there is some evidence of differences in physical findings between the malnourished WW II European theater prisoners and all other European theater POWs. Looking first at the broad ICD disease groups, one sees an appreciably higher lifetime prevalence rate of other endocrine diseases (which include the nutritional disorders). Moving to the selected set of medical conditions noted in similar studies of VA examinations of POWs, one sees appreciably higher lifetime prevalence rates of dysentery, beriberi, and frozen feet, all presumably the earlier sequelae of captivity. There are, in addition, appreciably higher rates of gastroenteritis—noninfectious gastroenteritis and colitis, but not irritable bowel syndrome—and of peripheral nerve disease, concentrated in the three categories of mononeuritis of the upper and lower limbs and hereditary and idiopathic peripheral neuropathy.

This chapter portrays most clearly the persistence and predominance of psychological aftereffects, now four-and-a-half decades after repatriation in some cases. Surely, posttraumatic stress disorder and depressive symptoms, both of particular interest and the focus of special data collection, are the most striking sequelae, and the findings from the symptom checklist suggest that many other psychological conditions are also much more prevalent among POWs than among their comparable controls. Physical findings are not nearly as striking, and earlier differences among POW groups may have lessened over the past 25 years. The special group of malnourished WW II European theater prisoners, however, exhibits not only elevated prevalence rates of conditions clearly linked with their earlier captivity, such as dysentery and beriberi, but also some apparently longer-term aftereffects, such as gastroenteritis and peripheral nerve disease.

The relative deficiency of apparent physical findings across the whole of the examined POW population, however, may be somewhat attributed to the relative paucity of specific a priori medical hypotheses. The analyses of Chapter 6 attempt to remedy this deficiency and focus more sharply on the source of current POW health problems by examining their associations with experiences in military captivity.

TABLE 5.E.2 Number and Lifetime Rate (per hundred) of Selected Neurological Diagnoses from the Medical Examination, for PWEM and PWE

	PWEM (*N*=83)		PWE (*N*=142)	
Diagnostic Category (ICD Code[a])	Number	Rate	Number	Rate
Trigeminal nerve disorders (350)	0	0.0	1	0.7
Facial nerve disorders (351)	0	0.0	1	0.7
Disorders of other cranial nerves (352)	1	1.2	0	0.0
Nerve root and plexus disorders (353)	0	0.0	1	0.7
Mononeuritis of upper limb and mononeuritis multiplex (354)	5	6.0	3	2.1
Mononeuritis of lower limb (355)	5	6.0	4	2.8
Hereditary and idiopathic peripheral neuropathy (356)	3	3.6	2	1.4
Inflammatory and toxic neuropathy (357)	1	1.2	1	0.7
Myoneural disorders (358)	0	0.0	0	0.0
Muscular dystrophies and other myopathies (359)	1	1.2	0	0.0

PWEM, prisoner of war, malnourished, European theater, WW II; PWE, prisoner of war, European theater, WW II.

[a]Coded to the ninth revision, International Classification of Diseases, Clinical Modification.

REFERENCES

Beebe GW. 1975. Follow-up studies of World War II and Korean war prisoners: II. Morbidity, disability, and maladjustments. Am. J. Epidemiol. 101:400-422.

Dent OF, Tennant CC, Goulston KJ. 1987. Precursors of depression in World War II veterans 40 years after the war. J. Nerv. Ment. Dis. 175:486-490.

Eberly RE, Engdahl BE. 1991. Prevalence of somatic and psychiatric disorders among former prisoners of war. Hosp. Commun. Psychiatry 42:807-813.

Goulston KJ, Dent OF, Chapuis PH, et al. 1985. Gastrointestinal morbidity among World War II prisoners of war: 40 years on. Med. J. Aust. 143:6-10.

Nefzger MD. 1970. Follow-up studies of World War II and Korean war prisoners: I. Study plan and mortality findings. Am. J. Epidemiol. 91:123-138.

Oboler S. 1987. American prisoners of war—an overview. In Williams T (ed.), Post-traumatic Stress Disorders: A Handbook for Clinicians. 1987. Disabled American Veterans, Cincinnati, pp. 131-143.

Tennant C, Goulston K, Dent O. 1986. The psychological effects of being a prisoner of war: forty years after release. Am. J. Psychiatry 143:618-621.

6

Further Analyses of Examination Data

The analyses undertaken in Chapter 5 were all directed at those issues that had been identified as important before the examination study actually began. By and large, they were simple, straightforward comparisons of POW and control disease prevalence rates. Unfortunately, while these are the most usual and orthodox types of analyses, they have their problems, both medical and statistical. In the hope that some of the inherent shortcomings of those analyses might be overcome, this chapter presents other analyses of the examination and psychological data, all of which lie outside the scope of the narrowly defined, formal assessments of Chapter 5. As noted earlier, the disappointingly low response rates for the exam render the customary statistical testing and inferences inappropriate. Thus, as in earlier chapters, statistical tests, when used, will merely provide an indication of "noteworthy" or "appreciable" differences or associations and not of statistically significant differences.

Aside from the difficulties caused by low response rates, the chief problem in Chapter 5 was the lack of definite, specific hypotheses about medical conditions, a lack easily seen when such conditions were contrasted with mental disorders. As explained earlier, similar research on former Australian prisoners of the Japanese, conducted on an admittedly smaller scale, found no excess prevalence of medical conditions among former POWs except for ulcer—specifically, a *history* of and *not current* ulcers—and increased use of analgesics, suggesting an increased prevalence of arthritis that was, however, not directly observable. The reasonable choice then was to look at broad disease categories, so as not to miss any important findings that might manifest themselves in the examination data. The danger of doing the same kind of analyses on a detailed level arises from the fact that doing literally thousands of statistical tests has the real risk of marking as a medical problem that which is merely statistical noise. This chapter attempts to gain a middle ground by revisiting and expanding the analyses in Chapter 4. Only a limited number of medical conditions will be considered in more detail, and the medical conditions to be studied will be chosen based on published epidemiological research and clinical material. To avoid a bias from historical reporting, only unresolved medical conditions will be discussed.

The core set of conditions included in Table 6.1 come from Eberly and Engdahl's study (see Chapter 4). All but one of the remaining conditions were chosen for analysis based on the published work of Oboler and subsequent personal communications (discussed under question E in Chapter 5). Thus, the conditions to be studied further were all suggested by epidemiologic or clinical considerations, and their selection was not based on examination findings, with one exception—fewer blood dyscrasias (discussed below).

In Chapter 4, an appreciably lower lifetime prevalence of diseases of the blood was noted, and in question C in Chapter 5 an examination of current prevalence data produced a similar finding. There were additional International Classification of Diseases rubrics with higher POW current prevalence rates as well, but in almost all of those cases, a specific disease had already been singled out for analysis—for example, ulcer in the digestive disease group and peripheral nerve disease in the nervous system group. The apparent deficit of other endocrine disease among PWP, which was primarily due to an excess number of WP cases of other metabolic and immunity disorders, is not analyzed further, given the earlier data on the possible nonrepresentativeness of the WP group and the failure of other control groups to show this excess.

The appreciably lower prevalence of blood diseases, however, is both persistent, appearing in both the lifetime and current prevalences derived from exam data, and pervasive, occurring in both the PWP and PWK groups as well as the PWE and PWEM, although in the latter the differences were not noteworthy. Moreover, the reason for this lower prevalence appears to be fairly specific, in that most of the deficit can be attributed to anemia, by and large "other and unspecified." All of these factors together argue for the inclusion of anemia in subsequent analyses; thus, although this is a condition suggested from examination of the data and *less* frequently found in POWs, it is nevertheless included in Table 6.1.

Table 6.1 presents data on the selected conditions for all study groups. As seen in Chapter 5, psychiatric illnesses predominate, with appreciably

TABLE 6.1 Prevalence Rates (percentages) of Medical and Psychiatric Diagnoses Among POWs, Unresolved Conditions Only, by Study Group

Diagnosis	PWP	PWE	PWEM	PWK	WP	WE	WK
Medical conditions							
Hypertension	50.8	41.6	49.4	38.0	37.0	37.0	40.8
Diabetes mellitus	14.8	13.4	12.1	12.5	18.5	7.4	10.7
Anemia	6.8[a]	7.0	4.8	5.2[a]	20.4[a]	11.1	18.5[a]
Cerebrovascular disease	1.6	1.4	2.4	2.2	0.0	0.0	2.9
Ischemic heart disease	27.2	23.9	27.7[a]	12.5	24.1	7.4[a]	16.5
Myocardial infarction	2.8	0.0	6.0	0.8	0.0	0.0	1.0
Intermittent claudication	17.2	9.2	14.5	13.2	11.1	3.7	6.8
Arterial vascular disease	33.2	23.9	30.1	23.3	27.8	29.6	18.5
Asthma	7.6	7.8	2.4	3.9	3.7	0.0	1.0
COPD	16.4	14.8	14.5	14.0	20.4	14.8	10.7
Peripheral nerve disease	20.4[a]	6.3	15.7	14.0[a]	7.4[a]	7.4	3.9[a]
Deafness	53.6	50.0	51.8	50.3	59.3	48.2	57.3
Ulcer	12.0	12.0	16.9	20.6[a]	13.0	7.4	4.9[a]
Gastroenteritis	14.4	13.4	24.1[a]	17.2[a]	5.6	3.7[a]	1.9[a]
Dysentery	0.4	0.0	2.4	1.2	0.0	0.0	0.0
Osteoarthritis	26.4	33.8	32.5	28.4	29.6	22.2	19.4
Traumatic arthritis	1.6	0.0	1.2	1.0	0.0	0.0	0.0
Malaria	0.8[a]	0.0	0.0	0.3	11.1[a]	0.0	1.0
Beriberi	0.0	0.0	0.0	0.3	0.0	0.0	0.0
Frozen feet	0.0	0.7	3.6	0.0	0.0	0.0	0.0
Psychiatric conditions							
Depressive disorder	46.8[a]	31.7[a]	50.6[a]	51.0[a]	13.0[a]	0.0[a]	22.3[a]
Bipolar I or II disorder	0.8	0.0	0.0	0.3	0.8	0.0	0.0
Alcohol abuse or dependence	12.8	14.1	19.3	27.5	14.8	7.4	32.0
Schizophrenia	1.2	0.0	2.4	3.2	0.0	0.0	1.0
PTSD	40.0[a]	20.4	27.7[a]	37.0[a]	0.0[a]	7.4[a]	10.7[a]
Generalized anxiety	38.8[a]	39.4[a]	55.4[a]	54.2[a]	9.3[a]	7.4[a]	22.3[a]
Number in sample	250	142	83	408	54	27	103

PWP, prisoner of war, Pacific theater, WW II; PWE, prisoner of war, European theater, WW II; PWEM, prisoner of war, malnourished, European theater, WW II; PWK, prisoner of war, Korean conflict; WP, war veteran, Pacific theater, WW II; WE, war veteran, European theater, WW II; WK, wounded war veteran, Korean conflict; COPD, chronic obstructive pulmonary disease; PTSD, posttraumatic stress disorder.

[a]Noteworthy (see text) difference between POW and control prevalence rates.

higher rates of depressive symptoms and generalized anxiety in POWs in all study groups; posttraumatic stress disorder (PTSD) rates are appreciably higher for all but PWE. Among the medical conditions, there are appreciably higher prevalence rates of ischemic heart disease for PWEM, peripheral nerve disease for PWP and PWK, and gastroenteritis for PWEM and PWK;

WP had an appreciably higher rate of malaria than PWP, but, again, doubts about the soundness of the findings from the WP group motivated the decision to conduct no further analyses. In addition, there were somewhat higher rates for hypertension in PWP, ischemic heart disease in PWE, intermittent claudication in PWK, gastroenteritis in PWP, and osteoarthritis in PWK.

Besides the problem of diagnostic categorization, there are other, statistical problems with the analyses of Chapter 5. First and foremost is the problem of control groups. The small samples in the control groups directly reflect their lower response rates, and although the demographic and VA hospitalization data in Chapter 3 were somewhat reassuring, it should be noted that the members of the WP group with completed exams, in particular, appear unusual. Among the three control groups, after eliminating the four medical conditions with zero prevalence rates, WP have the highest prevalence rates for 11 of the 15 remaining conditions. The WP group also has the only control prevalence rate—that for malaria—that is higher than a corresponding POW rate.

Second, there is the question of whether there are more statistically sensitive analyses that could be undertaken than those that simply compare POW versus control prevalence rates. Comparing POWs with themselves, using those less harshly treated as a basis for comparison with those more harshly treated, should not only provide a more sensitive analysis but should also avoid the problems that arise from analyzing data from a small and potentially unrepresentative control group, such as the WP.

This chapter continues with a set of analyses that use POWs as *internal controls* to provide independent information about possible associations between selected medical conditions and prior military captivity. The underlying idea is straightforward. Although the widest differences among subjects are thought to be between POWs and controls, there is sufficient variation among POWs to compare those who reported less harsh treatment in captivity with those reporting harsher treatment; this essentially uses the first group as an internal control for the second.

The overwhelming advantage of internal controls, although it may not be immediately obvious, is that one may include in the analyses any supplemental data collected only from POWs. This is particularly important in instances in which captivity data are present in such detail that a gradient for harshness of treatment can be established; if the prevalence of a particular medical condition then increases in a regular fashion with the increase in the harshness of treatment gradient, causality arguments are strengthened. The disadvantages of using internal controls include the possibility of reporting bias in the supplemental data collected only among POWs and lack of a true baseline, which would tend to underestimate the adverse effects of military captivity. In addition, the careful demographic balances between

POWs and controls that were established when the samples were taken are lost (although it is unclear how great a disadvantage this might be). Finally, because the PWEM group was not included in the 1967 follow-up and thus lacks the more detailed data on harshness of captivity, their examination data are not included in this chapter; there are, therefore, three study groups that are considered: PWP, PWE, and PWK.

Characterizing the harshness of treatment is the *sine qua non* of analyses that use internal controls. Clearly, a complete, simple characterization is impossible, and so one approximates. Even if there were available data characterizing the harshness of treatment in individual prison camps, their use would not be straightforward; for example, tracking an individual's movements in and out of various camps might prove to be fairly complicated. Furthermore, even if this exercise were successful, it is not clear whether aggregate prison camp data would adequately characterize the treatment of each and every individual POW. Instead, two kinds of military captivity data, each collected on an individual basis, are examined in this chapter: medical symptoms reported while in captivity and self-reported weight loss during captivity (both kinds of data were collected as part of Beebe's [1975] follow-up study). Weight loss during military captivity, in particular, is one of the strongest overall markers of severity of trauma and has been strongly associated with severity of aftereffects in published reports.

Medical symptom data regarding infectious and nutritional diseases during captivity were collected in 1965–1967 by a questionnaire sent to all POWs (not including PWEM). The POWs were given a checklist of physical conditions and asked to indicate, condition by condition, whether they suffered from the effects of a particular condition during captivity. These prison camp symptoms are listed in Table 6.2. In collecting symptom data by questionnaire, one encounters the possibility of recall bias; that is, persons with health problems at the time that the questionnaire is being filled out may be more likely to recall earlier harsh treatment than persons who were not ill at the time of data collection. The fact that these symptom data were collected some 25 years ago, however, removes the possibility of current recall bias—any recall bias must be associated with symptoms and medical conditions reported at the time of the earlier questionnaire.

The symptoms shown in Table 6.2 include many that are associated with nutritional deprivation. Later in this chapter, these prison camp symptoms will be aggregated into three separate measures, two of which—edema and visual symptoms (such as night blindness)—have obvious associations with specific nutritional deprivations (thiamin and vitamin A, respectively). Unfortunately, roughly one-quarter of the queried POWs did not provide data on weight loss or prison camp symptoms, and for the remainder of the chapter, those with missing data for these variables are excluded from the analyses.

TABLE 6.2 Prison Camp Symptoms Reported by Former POWs in the 1967 Follow-up Study

Malaria
Diarrhea lasting one week or more
Blood and mucus in stool
Amebic dysentery diagnosed by a physician
Swelling of lower limbs
Swelling in feet or ankles, or legs as a whole
Persistent difficulty seeing in the dark
Continuous pain or burning in eyes
Blurred vision
Eye pain in bright light
Loss of vision, one or both eyes
Red, raw scrotum
Deep cracks, corner of mouth
Persistent, severe sunburn
Red, swollen, bleeding gums
Soreness of tongue interfering with eating
Painful feet
Pain in leg muscles when squeezed
Cramps in feet and legs
Enlarged breasts

Table 6.3 shows prevalence rates of selected conditions for all PWP, PWE, and PWK combined and subdivided into two categories: those whose prison camp weight loss was 35% or less and those with more than 35% weight loss (this categorization was chosen to correspond with Engdahl's analyses). Because the prevalence rates in this chapter are all based on unresolved conditions, the rates for dysentery, malaria, beriberi, and frozen feet, all presumably short-term sequelae of captivity, were very low; therefore, these conditions, as well as bipolar disorder, were removed from further consideration.

The data in Table 6.3 show a number of noteworthy differences in prevalence rates between low- and high-weight-loss groups, including intermittent claudication, arterial vascular disease, peripheral nerve disease, and osteoarthritis. In the light of the findings discussed in earlier chapters, this appreciable association of weight loss and intermittent claudication and peripheral nerve disease is probably not surprising, nor are the appreciably higher rates of depressive disorder and PTSD among the high-weight-loss group; Eberly and Engdahl's study showed significant associations with depression, schizophrenia, PTSD, and generalized anxiety disorder. However, the inverse association of osteoarthritis and weight loss—*less* osteoar-

TABLE 6.3 Prevalence Rates (percentages) of Medical and Psychiatric Diagnoses Among POWs, by Percent Body Weight Loss During Captivity

	Body Weight Loss	
Diagnosis	35% or Less (*N*=281)	More than 35% (*N*=287)
Medical conditions		
Hypertension	43.4	43.6
Diabetes mellitus	11.4	14.6
Anemia	5.3	5.6
Cerebrovascular disease	1.4	1.7
Ischemic heart disease	19.6	21.3
Myocardial infarction	0.7	1.1
Intermittent claudication	10.3	17.4[a]
Arterial vascular disease	21.0	31.4[a]
Asthma	5.0	5.9
COPD	12.5	17.1
Peripheral nerve disease	10.7	19.2[a]
Deafness	48.8	55.8
Ulcer	15.0	17.8
Gastroenteritis	15.7	20.6
Osteoarthritis	34.9	25.8[a]
Traumatic arthritis	0.7	1.4
Psychiatric conditions		
Depressive disorder	40.2	53.7[a]
Alcohol abuse or dependence	19.6	19.9
Schizophrenia	3.2	2.1
PTSD	29.2	41.5[a]
Generalized anxiety	44.5	51.2

COPD, chronic obstructive pulmonary disease; PTSD, posttraumatic stress disorder.

[a]Noteworthy (see text) difference between prevalence rates.

thritis in the *higher* weight loss group—is the first such finding of its type in this report.

Table 6.4 contains data on the same medical conditions that are noted in Table 6.3, but this table shows associations with the number of reported prison camp symptoms. In this analysis, self-reported conditions were simply added together, and all POW respondents were arranged into three categories: those reporting 0 to 3 conditions, those reporting 4 to 9 conditions, and those reporting 10 or more conditions. There are a number of conditions in which prevalence rates rise from the lowest symptom category to the middle category, and then to the high category. Rather than merely look

TABLE 6.4 Prevalence Rates (percentages) of Medical and Psychiatric Diagnoses Among POWs, by Number of Prison Camp Symptoms

	Number of Prison Camp Symptoms		
Diagnosis	0 to 3 (N=165)	4 to 9 (N=240)	10 or more (N=185)
Medical conditions			
Hypertension	44.9	42.5	43.2
Diabetes mellitus	14.6	9.6	14.6
Anemia	6.7	5.8	4.3
Cerebrovascular disease	0.6	2.9	0.5
Ischemic heart disease	15.8	19.6	23.8
Myocardial infarction	0.6	0.0	2.2
Intermittent claudication	9.1	13.8	18.4[a]
Arterial vascular disease	22.4	24.2	31.9[a]
Asthma	3.0	5.0	8.1[a]
COPD	12.1	13.8	17.3
Peripheral nerve disease	9.7	12.9	21.1[a]
Deafness	49.1	54.6	50.8
Ulcer	10.3	22.1	14.1
Gastroenteritis	14.6	17.1	20.5
Osteoarthritis	33.9	30.8	24.9
Traumatic arthritis	1.2	0.0	2.2
Psychiatric conditions			
Depressive disorder	32.7	44.6	61.1[a]
Alcohol abuse or dependence	15.8	22.9	18.9
Schizophrenia	0.6	2.5	4.3[a]
PTSD	23.0	38.8	40.0[a]
Generalized anxiety	40.0	48.3	52.4[a]

COPD, chronic obstructive pulmonary disease; PTSD, posttraumatic stress disorder.

[a]Noteworthy (see text) difference among prevalence rates.

for differences among the three categories, the prevalence rates in Table 6.4 were subjected to a chi-square test for linear trend, which indicates increasing or decreasing linear relationships between symptom category and prevalence rate. Although the results of these tests, like the others in this report, cannot be used as the basis for valid statistical inferences, they are more powerful than the usual chi-square test and may thus generate new hypotheses regarding associations of disease and prison camp treatment.

Among the medical conditions, there is a noteworthy linear increase in prevalence as symptoms increase; see, for example, intermittent claudication, arterial vascular disease, asthma, and peripheral nerve disease. Similar noteworthy associations hold for depressive disorder, schizophrenia, PTSD, and generalized anxiety. There are also fairly strong relationships between symptom category and ischemic heart disease, myocardial infarction, and osteoarthritis, although the prevalence of unresolved osteoarthritis *falls* with increasing past reporting of prison camp symptoms. This last finding is consistent with the earlier finding of an inverse association with weight loss.

Although the data on weight loss and prison camp symptoms are more easily viewed when categorized as in Tables 6.3 and 6.4, their actual values can be used to calculate product-moment correlations, treating each medical condition as a "zero-one" value (i.e., either absent [0] or present [1] for each examined subject). The results of this analysis are shown in Table 6.5, with separate columns for weight loss and symptoms correlations for each of the three study groups.

Many of the appreciable correlations in Table 6.5 reflect earlier noteworthy differences in the combined POW data in Tables 6.3 and 6.4. The noteworthy association of prison camp symptoms with peripheral nerve disease, for example, is seen in both PWP and PWE, and all three groups show appreciable correlations of prison camp symptoms with depressive disorder. Some conditions, however, have noteworthy associations in only one POW group: intermittent claudication (PWK), arterial vascular disease (PWK), asthma (PWP), PTSD (PWK), and generalized anxiety (PWP). One condition, schizophrenia, showed no appreciable association in any of the three individual groups. Part of the explanation for the sparser findings among the individual groups is no doubt a result of their smaller sample sizes. Similar comments apply to the correlations with weight loss, except that only arterial vascular disease among the medical conditions shows a noteworthy correlation in more than one group.

This last observation points up one of the shortcomings in the data in Tables 6.3 and 6.4. Both tables were generated by pooling the data from all three POW groups (PWP, PWE, and PWK); therefore, some of the apparent associations between weight loss and symptom categories might actually be due to underlying differences among POW groups in harshness of treatment (and thus amount of weight loss and number of prison camp symptoms). Moreover, if weight loss and symptoms are markers for the POW group, the potential exists for some confounding between them and age, since PWK are notably younger than PWP and PWE.

Looking at each POW group separately, as in Table 6.5, removes the possibility of confounding group and weight loss or prison camp symptom effects, but it has its own drawbacks. Chief among these is the reduced sample size, which may mean that possibly noteworthy associations are lost in statistical "noise." One way to examine the effects of weight loss and prison camp symptoms while controlling for the separate effect of POW

TABLE 6.5 Correlations of Rates of Medical and Psychiatric Diagnoses Among POWs with Number of Prison Camp Symptoms and Percent Weight Loss

	PWP		PWK		PWE	
Diagnosis	Prison Camp Symptoms (*N*=189)	Weight Loss (*N*=187)	Prison Camp Symptoms (*N*=286)	Weight Loss (*N*=275)	Prison Camp Symptoms (*N*=115)	Weight Loss (*N*=106)
Medical conditions						
Hypertension	.025	–.028	–.068	.021	.009	.119
Diabetes mellitus	.023	.073	.058	.064	–.176	–.112
Anemia	–.059	–.010	–.050	–.071	–.107	–.001
Cerebrovascular disease	–.025	.079	–.041	–.037	.065	.060
Ischemic heart disease	.073	.012	.109	.073	.066	.178
Myocardial infarction	.054	.013	–.109	.061	N.a.	N.a.
Intermittent claudication	.076	.112	.125[a]	.105	–.064	.169
Arterial vascular disease	.068	.108	.119[a]	.120[a]	–.153	.216[a]
Asthma	.149[a]	.154[a]	.077	.077	.062	–.079
COPD	.065	.033	.047	.042	.019	.170
Peripheral nerve disease	.192[a]	.075	.001	.037	.184[a]	.259[a]
Deafness	.055	.110	–.045	.039	–.098	.066
Ulcer	.031	–.022	.062	.025	.182	.179
Gastroenteritis	.085	.119	.080	.038	.126	–.088
Osteoarthritis	.134	–.124	–.114	–.041	.105	.035
Traumatic arthritis	.105	.105	.012	.040	N.a.	N.a.
Psychiatric conditions						
Depressive disorder	.313[a]	.132	.155[a]	.050	.192[a]	–.025
Alcohol abuse or dependence	.056	.082	.040	.060	–.013	.060
Schizophrenia	.030	.083	.051	–.150[a]	N.a.	N.a.
PTSD	.079	–.004	.122[a]	.113	.024	.139
Generalized anxiety	.279[a]	.144[a]	.073	–.014	–.018	–.019

PWP, prisoner of war, Pacific theater, WW II; PWK, prisoner of war, Korean conflict; PWE, prisoner of war, European theater, WW II; COPD, chronic obstructive pulmonary disease; PTSD, posttraumatic stress disorder; N.a., not applicable.

[a]Noteworthy (see text) correlation.

group is to perform a Cochran-Mantel-Haenszel (CMH) analysis, which estimates the common association between a given medical condition and a weight or symptom score, using separate data for each POW group. This kind of analysis requires an assumption that the data in the separate POW groups are homogeneous, which can be tested, and provides a single summary estimate of the strength of association.

A CMH analysis was conducted for all of the selected medical conditions used in previously reported analyses in this chapter; only the noteworthy results are displayed in Table 6.6. Shown in the table are results based on an analysis of the risk ratio (which is akin to a ratio of prevalence rates) for the weight loss data (which have two categories—see Table 6.3) and a measure of general association for the prison camp symptom data (which have three categories—see Table 6.4). All noteworthy associations are so designated; a few less marked associations are also shown.

The data in Table 6.6 present a picture similar to earlier findings, even with the statistical adjustment for the effect of POW group differences. There are noteworthy associations between weight loss and arterial vascular disease, depressive disorder, and PTSD, and important but less strong associations between weight loss and intermittent claudication, peripheral nerve disease, and osteoarthritis. (Again, the latter is an association between *higher* weight loss and a *lower* prevalence of unresolved osteoarthritis.) The data for symptom scores show noteworthy associations with ischemic heart disease, ulcer, asthma, depressive disorder, and generalized anxiety, as well as somewhat weaker associations with PTSD and cerebrovascular disease.

That there are a number of common medical conditions among different analyses is a comforting finding; it suggests that the analyses undertaken thus far in this chapter have unearthed a number of strong candidates for current medical conditions that might be associated with earlier military captivity. As a final refinement, statistical analyses were undertaken to determine the joint, simultaneous effects of weight loss and prison camp symptoms, taking into account the differences among POW groups.

TABLE 6.6 Medical Conditions with a High Risk Ratio or General Association Between Body Weight Loss During Captivity or Prison Camp Symptoms, Adjusted for POW Group Differences

Risk Ratio for Weight Loss (N=568)	General Association with Prison Camp Symptoms (N=590)
Intermittent claudication	Cerebrovascular disease
Arterial vascular disease[a]	Ischemic heart disease[a]
Peripheral neuropathy	Ulcer[a]
Osteoarthritis	Asthma[a]
Depressive disorder[a]	Depressive disorder[a]
PTSD[a]	PTSD
	Generalized anxiety[a]

PSTD, posttraumatic stress disorder.

[a]Noteworthy (see text) association.

For this analysis, the prison camp symptom data were further refined along the lines of Beebe's previous work (1975). Specifically, reported symptoms on edema (two items: feet or ankle and leg swelling) were combined into a single marker of edema; reported visual symptoms (five items) were combined into a single variable that counts the number of these responses (from zero to five); and the remaining 13 symptoms were added together for a third symptom marker. These three symptom markers plus percent weight loss and POW group were used as independent variables in logistic regression analyses of the medical conditions reported in Table 6.6, plus schizophrenia (from Tables 6.4 and 6.5) and gastroenteritis (from Table 6.1). The use of logistic regression not only enables independent estimates of the effects of weight loss and the three symptom scores to be made, but also permits the analysis of all the available data at one time while controlling for differences among the three POW groups. The latter is accomplished by creating two variables, one comparing PWP with PWE and one comparing PWK with PWE, and including them in the regression. Backward stepwise regressions were fit to eliminate those variables without appreciable associations, although in some cases in which no independent variables were appreciably associated with a condition, additional regressions were fit using variables with less strong associations.

Table 6.7 shows the results of these logistic regressions for all of the medical conditions noted above. Estimates of odds ratios are shown together with 95% confidence limits; confidence limits that do not include the value 1.0 would be considered to have a noteworthy association with a particular medical condition. Odds ratios greater than 1.0 indicate that a higher prevalence is associated with the factor, while odds ratios of less than 1.0 indicate a lower prevalence. For example, ischemic heart disease is 1.737 times *more* likely to be found among POWs who reported symptoms of edema than among POWs who did not, and it is 0.405 times *less* likely to be found among PWK, compared with PWE.

In the cases of visual and other symptoms, the estimates of risk are for a single reported symptom, and the effects of more than one symptom are multiplicative. For example, each additional reported other symptom raises the estimate of the odds of having intermittent claudication by 1.11; 2 reported symptoms raise the odds to 1.23, 3 to 1.37, and so forth, up to a maximum of 13, for which the risk is 3.93 (1.1109^{13}) times as high as for those with no reported symptoms. The situation is similar for percent weight loss, and here the odds ratio associated with a 10% weight loss is reported in Table 6.7. Odds ratios for other values of weight loss can be easily calculated from these figures.

Among the nonpsychiatric conditions, all but cerebrovascular disease and osteoarthritis have a noteworthy association with one or more markers of harshness of treatment during captivity. For cerebrovascular disease,

TABLE 6.7 Odds Ratios for the Current Prevalence of Selected Medical Conditions, by Important Predictive Factors (N=546)

	Important Predictors[a]		
Diagnosis	Factor	Odds Ratio	95% Confidence Interval
Medical conditions			
Ischemic heart disease	Edema	1.737	(1.092–2.762)
	PWK	0.405	(0.259–0.635)
Cerebrovascular disease	Visual symptoms	1.735	(0.874–3.445)
Intermittent claudication	Percent wt. loss	1.311	(1.032–1.664)
	Other symptoms	1.111	(1.014–1.217)
Arterial vascular disease	Percent wt. loss	1.389	(1.180–1.635)
	PWK	0.606	(0.406–0.903)
Peripheral nerve disease	Edema	2.365	(1.372–4.077)
Ulcer	Visual symptoms	1.152	(0.996–1.333)
	PWK	1.801	(1.137–2.853)
Gastroenteritis	Other symptoms	1.074	(1.002–1.152)
Osteoarthritis	Percent wt. loss	0.879	(0.764–1.011)
Asthma	Visual symptoms	1.288	(1.032–1.607)
	PWK	0.514	(0.240–1.010)
Psychiatric conditions			
Depressive disorder	Other symptoms	1.176	(1.110–1.246)
Schizophrenia	PWK	4.395	(1.226–15.753)
Posttraumatic stress disorder	Visual symptoms	1.146	(1.015–1.293)
	PWP	2.431	(1.318–4.481)
	PWK	2.350	(1.309–4.219)
Generalized anxiety	Other symptoms	1.097	(1.037–1.161)
	PWK	2.144	(1.517–3.030)

PWK, prisoner of war, Korean conflict; PWP, prisoner of war, Pacific theater, WW II; PWE, prisoner of war, European theater, WW II; WP, war veteran, Pacific theater, WW II. Factors included in the analyses are as follows: **percent weight loss** shows the risk for each 10% of reported weight loss; **edema** is the presence or absence of swelling in legs or feet and ankles; **visual symptoms** are 0 to 5 of the following—persistent difficulty seeing in the dark, continuous pain or burning in the eyes; blurred vision, eye pain in bright light, or loss of vision in one or both eyes; **other symptoms** are a count of remaining symptoms in Table 6.2. There are two independent group comparisons: **PWP** compares PWP with PWE, and **PWK** compares PWK with PWE.

[a]Not all factors showed noteworthy associations with outcomes.

there is the suggestion of an association with visual symptoms, and for osteoarthritis, a similar association with percent weight loss: both of these give evidence of the presence of potentially important but weaker associations. No one symptom marker predominates in its associations with unresolved medical conditions; rather, each shows only one or two noteworthy associations.

All psychiatric conditions have some noteworthy association with a prison camp symptom marker except for schizophrenia, which is appreciably higher in PWK and has a weaker strong association with other prison camp symptoms. Except for PTSD, which shows appreciable differences between PWP and PWE as well as PWE and PWK, the only noteworthy group differences involve the PWE versus PWK comparison.

To summarize, this chapter's analyses were directed at more specific medical conditions and, using POWs as internal controls, have suggested a number of new findings. Appreciably higher prevalences of current ischemic heart disease, intermittent claudication, arterial vascular disease, peripheral nerve disease, ulcer, and asthma appear to be associated with nutritional deprivation and other measures of treatment during imprisonment; there are less strong associations of these factors with current prevalence of gastroenteritis as well as an apparently lower prevalence of osteoarthritis in those with higher weight loss.

The results of these analyses, however, are far from uniform in their findings of association, and the meaning of the different prison camp symptom markers is far from evident. Clearly, the customary POW-versus-control analyses and analyses that use internal POW controls yield complementary types of findings. In the next chapter, all of these findings are brought together in a comprehensive discussion.

REFERENCE

Beebe GW. 1975. Follow-up studies of World War II and Korean war prisoners. II. Morbidity, disability, and maladjustments. Am. J. Epidemiol. 101:400-422.

7

Review of Data Quality and Study Findings

The creation of the medical examination survey, whose data form the basis of this report, was largely a matter of opportunity. Although data were available from repatriation exams, and questionnaire- and records-based investigations had provided four decades of follow-up data, no examination data had ever been collected from the entire, combined MFUA cohort of POWs and controls. It was not until the VA's POW protocol exam program began in 1983, largely as an outreach effort, that the opportunity to examine this large group of POWs (and later, controls) presented itself. The VA's POW program was the crucial factor in the design of this survey because it provided the extensive network of physicians and other health care professionals needed to collect the examination data. Moreover, because the program had already been begun as a clinical program, there would be no additional costs in using it for research purposes.

The VA's POW examination program had not, however, been designed for research use, and here the benefits of combining it with the MFUA's longitudinal study were manifest. The earliest directive from the VA concerning the research study, Circular 10-87-138, put it thus: "In order to adapt this [VA] program for research purposes, it is necessary to collect protocol examination data on representative groups of POWs rather than to analyze data for only men who have presented themselves for examination." It was not until later (as directed under a separate VA circular) that control groups were added, because the proposed inclusion of non-POW veterans in the VA's examination program posed some difficulties and therefore was not immediately accepted. Eventually, however, the arguments for the inclusion of non-POW controls were persuasive: it would further strengthen the research by providing important comparison data to help interpret the findings among POWs. In sum, the combination of the VA's POW outreach program and the MFUA's research program was designed to produce a research survey with the best features of both kinds of programs.

Yet the opportunity to apply the existing mechanisms of the VA examination program to the MFUA cohort was not without its accompanying drawbacks. For example, although the widespread network of VA medical facilities provided coast-to-coast geographic coverage, it came with a built-in lack of standardization of examination procedures. Despite the publication of VA directives, the actual conduct of examinations necessarily varied from place to place and from time to time, in part as a result of local administrative customs, but mostly because of the underlying variability among examiners in the way they performed a "typical" examination. The study thus lacked the common, rigidly specified procedures of many research protocols. Yet despite these limitations, a large mass of important examination data has been accumulated.

DATA QUALITY

Before discussing the analysis of these data, some discussion of their quality is in order. The overall rate of completed, coded examinations, reported in Chapter 3, was disappointingly low—around 40–50% in POWs and 10–14% in controls. Some of the large difference in POW and control examination rates, in itself disquieting, is due to the fact that a number of POWs, the so-called volunteers, came in for examinations before the formal research program began. Because the VA's POW examination program began in 1983 and the research study began in 1986, there was ample opportunity for this to occur.

In general, however, at least in the previous morbidity follow-ups in 1967 (Beebe, 1975) and 1984 (Page, 1988), it has been the case that control response rates were lower than POW response rates. As evidence for this general statement, the same disparity in POW and control response rates is again seen in their responses to the supplemental psychological questionnaire mailing sponsored by the National Institute of Mental Health: questionnaire response rates were 25–30% for POWs and only 10–25% for controls. Interestingly, only relatively minor differences are apparent among POW groups or among control groups, except for the Korean conflict POWs and controls. These groups each had the highest response rates among POWs and controls.

Chapter 3 also included brief comparisons of demographic aspects and VA hospitalization rates for respondents and nonrespondents. There were few appreciable demographic differences between POWs who completed exams and those eligible subjects who did not. Among those with completed exams were higher proportions of men with service in the Air Corps and with a higher level of education. WE respondents had a higher proportion of men who were single at entry into service and who had been inducted.

VA hospitalization data for subjects with completed exams, eligible subjects without completed exams, and ineligible subjects were obtained for 1969–1985, predating the examination survey; these data provide evidence from a separate source about differences among the three groups. There were no appreciable differences in VA hospitalization rates among the above three comparison categories in any of the POW or control groups. These data thus suggest no overwhelming differences in health, at least as it is measured by 26 years of VA hospitalization data, between respondents and nonrespondents.

It is not unusual to find differences between survey respondents and nonrespondents, typically on measures of education (Comstock and Helsing, 1973). In an earlier study of nonresponse bias for the 1984–1985 questionnaire follow-up, Page (1991) found that nonrespondents were generally older, less well educated, and of lower military rank; in addition, they had previously reported more prison camp symptoms and slightly less weight loss. Demographic data were then used to predict depressive symptoms, and it was shown that there were only small differences between observed scores for respondents and predicted scores for nonrespondents, suggesting that nonresponse bias was not a major factor. Although a similar analysis has not yet been undertaken for the examination data from this study, the lack of obvious nonresponse bias in the 1984–1985 questionnaire follow-up, together with a similar lack of such bias indicated in the demographic and VA hospitalization data, is somewhat reassuring.

CHAPTER-BY-CHAPTER REVIEW OF RESULTS

Perhaps the signal feature of the examination data collection is its magnitude—the 1,067 examinations provide diagnostic data on more than 65,000 coded medical conditions. These exam data provided the basis, in Chapter 4, for the calculation of lifetime prevalence rates—that is, the probability that a given person has ever had (or still has) some specified disease. According to the exam data, POWs had higher lifetime prevalences than controls for a number of medical conditions: infectious disease (PWK), endocrine disease other than diabetes (PWP and PWK), psychoses (all but PWP), neuroses (all), neurological disease (PWP and PWK), urogenital disease (PWE), injuries and poisonings (PWE and PWEM), acute respiratory disease (PWK), digestive disease (PWK), skin disease (PWK), and other symptoms (PWK). Both PWP and PWK had an appreciably *lower* lifetime prevalence of blood diseases. In general, however, prevalence levels were similar among POWs and not strikingly different, for the most part, from control rates.

Chapter 4 also introduced the first external comparison data, showing similar lifetime prevalence rates for selected conditions that were taken from Eberly and Engdahl's (1991) study of POW examinations at the Minneapolis Medical Center. In some instances, lifetime prevalence rates were quite comparable—for example, in the case of hypertension rates for all MFUA POWs, all Minneapolis POWs, all MFUA controls, and the general population. However, in several other cases—diabetes, myocardial infarction, and cerebrovascular accident—lifetime prevalence rates were apparently lower for Minneapolis POWs than for the three other groups. Even more obvious differences could be seen between prevalence rates for psychiatric conditions in the combined data for MFUA and Minneapolis POWs: rates for depression were apparently higher for MFUA POWs and rates of posttraumatic stress disorder (PTSD) lower.

Known differences in age, length of captivity, and harshness of treatment during captivity made it reasonable to examine lifetime prevalence data for MFUA POWs and controls and for Minneapolis POWs separately, by war theater. Table 4.4 displayed lifetime prevalence rates for selected Eberly and Engdahl diagnostic categories. The MFUA data showed a rough equality across POW groups for most of the conditions not directly linked to prison camp treatment (i.e., those other than dysentery, malaria, beriberi, and frozen feet). Indeed, in regard to medical conditions, most of the noteworthy differences between MFUA POWs and controls were concentrated in the categories of prison camp–related conditions, with hypertension (among PWP) and ulcer (among PWK) the only exceptions.

The Minneapolis POWs can also be compared with the MFUA POWs. MFUA POWs had notably higher rates for intermittent claudication (all groups) and dysentery (all groups), while the MFUA PWEM, who have no comparable Minneapolis POW group, also had higher rates of hypertension and frozen feet than the Minneapolis PWE. In addition, the MFUA PWK had higher lifetime prevalences than their Minneapolis counterparts for malaria, beriberi, and frozen feet. In summary, most of the striking differences between the MFUA and Minneapolis POWs were for prison camp–related conditions.

Compared with MFUA controls, MFUA POWs have appreciably higher lifetime prevalence rates of depressive disorder and generalized anxiety disorder (across all POW groups) and PTSD (for PWP and PWK only). MFUA POW rates are also uniformly higher than Minneapolis POW rates for depressive disorder; they are uniformly lower for PTSD and roughly equal for generalized anxiety disorder, with differences across war eras not as pronounced as for some medical conditions. Finally, among MFUA controls, the Korean combat veteran controls (WK) apparently have much higher psychiatric morbidity than other control groups. It is worth noting again that these Korean controls differ from the WW II controls in having been selected from a group of men who had been wounded and returned to action; the Chapter 4 data show that although they were not prisoners, WK probably have increased lifetime psychiatric morbidity as a result of their war experience.

Chapter 5 addressed five basic questions, each of which had been posed before the study began. These questions were based on the preliminary findings of the 1984–1985 questionnaire follow-up as well as on limited findings from other, published studies. Question A asked whether psychiatric illness was higher in POWs than in controls; the answer was that there were appreciably higher rates of illness for several specific psychiatric conditions. In particular, the rates for PTSD were appreciably higher in POWs measured independently in each of three different ways: examination, Structured Clinical Interview for DSM-III-R (SCID), or questionnaire (the Mississippi scale). Rates of depressive disorder were similarly elevated, again measured independently in three ways: examination, Center for Epidemiologic Studies depression scale (CES-D) questionnaire, or Beck questionnaire. The finding of an appreciably higher rate of PTSD was particularly important, in that the 1984–1985 survey results had led to a hypothesis that PTSD was an underlying psychiatric diagnosis or comorbid condition associated with high rates of depressive symptoms. Additional data from the 90-item Hopkins Symptom Check List (SCL-90), however, suggest that psychiatric illness is not necessarily limited to PTSD and depressive disorder. The SCL-90 showed a wide range of psychiatric pathology across many disparate indices, with appreciably higher POW scores on a global symptom index. Psychiatric illness was most pronounced in PWK, PWEM, and PWP groups.

Question B asked whether there were important differences among measurement instruments for psychiatric illness. The answer here was that there were noteworthy differences among the various ways of measuring PTSD and depressive disorder. For PTSD, the exam and structured clinical interview agreed much more closely with each other than with the questionnaire, which had been designed and tested among Vietnam-era combat veterans. For depressive disorder, one scale (the CES-D) gave appreciably higher estimates of depressive disorder (although this scale is in the strictest sense a symptom scale); the other, the Beck scale, gave estimates that were much closer to the rates of clinical diagnosis. In every case, however, there were noteworthy differences between POWs and controls, regardless of how psychiatric illness was measured.

Question C asked whether earlier hospitalization rates were comparable to recent rates of VA hospitalization. In general, the answer was that there were apparently fewer differences between POWs and controls now than in

1967. A comparison of lifetime and current prevalence rates from the present exam also showed that differences in morbidity appear to have lessened over time.

Question D asked whether examination and earlier self-reported questionnaire data provided comparable estimates of illness prevalence. The answer was that medical conditions were self-reported by questionnaire much less frequently than they were noted during examination; typically, self-reported prevalence was only one-half to one-tenth the examination-based value. Some of this disparity appeared to be the result of limitations in the questionnaire design, such as a fixed number of blanks for responses, as well as of differences between physicians and questionnaire respondents in the use of medical terminology.

Question E asked whether the special, albeit small, subset of severely malnourished European prisoners, PWEM, differed from their European theater counterparts, PWE. The answer was that PWEM had an appreciably higher lifetime prevalence of dysentery, beriberi, frozen feet, peripheral nerve disease, and gastroenteritis. The latter two conditions, which are not as clearly related to prison camp treatment as the former, were studied in further diagnostic detail. Higher PWEM rates (compared with PWE) of peripheral nerve disease were concentrated in three specific categories: mononeuritis of the upper limb, mononeuritis of the lower limb, and hereditary and idiopathic neuropathy. Higher rates of gastroenteritis in PWEM were accounted for almost entirely by noninfectious gastroenteritis and colitis and not by irritable bowel syndrome, which has already been presumptively linked to military captivity.

The results of the analyses in Chapter 5 showed that there continue to be psychological aftereffects of military captivity as long as 45 years after repatriation and that these psychological illnesses are still the most striking sequelae of military captivity among WW II and Korean conflict POWs. Less evidence was uncovered concerning nonpsychological aftereffects, possibly because these effects were not as pronounced but also perhaps because the medical conditions were analyzed in broad categories to avoid missing any important but unanticipated findings. The use of these broad categories rather than more specific ones was a choice dictated by the relative paucity of specific medical hypotheses formulated at the time the study was designed.

In Chapter 6, a different sort of analysis was undertaken to complement the analyses of Chapter 5. As a first step, a specific set of medical conditions was selected, based on published reports of POW examinations at two VA medical centers, Minneapolis and Denver; current (that is, unresolved) prevalence rates for these conditions for POWs and controls were then compared. This analysis showed higher rates for POWs for the following conditions: ischemic heart disease (PWEM only), peripheral nerve disease

(PWP and PWK), ulcer (PWK only), gastroenteritis (PWEM and PWK), depressive disorder (PWP, PWE, PWEM, and PWK), PTSD (PWP, PWEM, and PWK), and generalized anxiety disorder (PWP, PWE, PWEM, and PWK). With the exception of malaria (in which case PWP rates were *lower* than WP rates), conditions showing noteworthy differences in current prevalence between a POW and control group were included in the final stage of analysis (discussed below).

In the next step of the process, the selected conditions were subjected to a second screening analysis to determine whether the prevalence of any of these conditions was associated with the specific factors that measured harshness of treatment as a POW, such as percentage of body weight loss. These analyses necessarily compared POWs with one another, avoiding the problems of earlier analyses that used small control samples. The use of internal controls in this analysis was thought to be statistically sensitive, that is, more apt to identify an association between medical conditions and earlier POW experience.

The second set of screening analyses looked first at the simple associations between the prevalence of the selected medical conditions and percentage of body weight lost, as well as at associations of prevalence with the number of reported prison camp medical symptoms (see Table 6.2), an overall measure of severity of treatment. POWs who reported more than a 35% body weight loss had appreciably elevated prevalences of intermittent claudication, arterial vascular disease, peripheral nerve disease, depressive disorder, and PTSD; they also had a *lower* prevalence of osteoarthritis. POWs who reported more prison camp symptoms compared with other POWs had appreciably higher prevalences of intermittent claudication, arterial vascular disease, peripheral nerve disease, depressive disorder, PTSD, generalized anxiety, and schizophrenia.

When the data were analyzed separately by POW group and body weight and prison camp symptoms were treated as continuous (rather than stratified) measures, many of these associations persisted. In addition, others were seen: asthma (PWP), peripheral nerve disease (PWP and PWE), intermittent claudication (PWK), arterial vascular disease (PWK and PWE), depressive disorder (PWP, PWE, and PWK), schizophrenia (PWK), PTSD (PWK), and generalized anxiety (PWP). Finally, a preliminary multivariate analysis, analyzing all POW data jointly but controlling for the different POW groups, found intermittent claudication, arterial vascular disease, peripheral neuropathy, osteoarthritis, depressive disorder, and PTSD to be strongly associated with percent weight loss; it found cerebrovascular disease, ischemic heart disease, ulcer, asthma, depressive disorder, PTSD, and generalized anxiety disorder to be strongly associated with prison camp symptoms.

The final analysis comprised the medical and psychiatric conditions for which there were findings of either an appreciably higher prevalence in some POW group or a noteworthy association with some military captivity factor. The prevalence data for these conditions were reanalyzed using logistic regression to determine the joint effects of weight loss and prison camp symptoms; POW group differences were also taken into account. For this analysis, prison camp symptoms were further refined into three separate measures—the presence of edema, the number of visual symptoms (such as night blindness), and the number of other symptoms—and considered along with percent weight loss.

The logistic regression analyses showed that edema was associated with a higher prevalence of ischemic heart disease and peripheral nerve disease; visual symptoms were associated with higher prevalences of cerebrovascular disease, ulcers, asthma, and posttraumatic stress disorder; and other symptoms were associated with higher prevalences of intermittent claudication, gastroenteritis, depressive disorder, and generalized anxiety. Percent weight loss was associated with a higher prevalence of intermittent claudication and arterial vascular disease and strongly associated with a *lower* prevalence of osteoarthritis. In most cases the odds ratios, which estimate the size of the increased prevalences, were between 1.0 and 2.0, indicating relatively moderate elevations in prevalence. It should also be noted, however, that the estimated effects of visual and other symptoms increased gradually with each additional reported symptom. Thus, the cumulative effect on the relative odds for POWs with a large number of symptoms could be quite substantial.

The effects on prevalence of POW group, per se, were mostly limited to PWK, but PWP showed an appreciably elevated prevalence of PTSD, compared with PWE. For PWK, again compared with PWE, there were noteworthy associations with a higher prevalence of ulcer, PTSD, schizophrenia, and generalized anxiety, and noteworthy associations with a *lower* prevalence of ischemic heart disease, arterial vascular disease, and asthma. These latter associations with lower prevalences appear to be related to age.

REFERENCES

Beebe GW. 1975. Follow-up studies of World War II and Korean war prisoners. II. Morbidity, disability, and maladjustments. Am. J. Epidemiol. 101:400-422.

Comstock GW, Helsing KJ. 1973. Characteristics of respondents and nonrespondents to a questionnaire for estimating community mood. Am. J. Epidemiol. 97:233-239.

Eberly RE, Engdahl BE. 1991. Prevalence of somatic and psychiatric disorders among former prisoners of war. Hosp. Commun. Psychiatry 42:807-813.

Page WF. 1988. A Report of the Longitudinal Follow-up of Former Prisoners of War of World War II and the Korean Conflict: Data on Depressive Symptoms from the 1984–1985 Questionnaire. Final report to the Veterans Administration under contract V101(93)P-1088. Medical Follow-up Agency, Institute of Medicine. Washington, DC.

Page WF. 1991. Using longitudinal data to estimate nonresponse bias. Soc. Psychiatry Psychiatr. Epidemiol. 26:127-131.

8

Literature Review and Further Discussion of Findings

The wealth of findings from the preceding chapters are most easily brought together and discussed when organized by disease. This chapter also reviews other pertinent literature and relates it, by organ system, to the disease-specific examination findings noted earlier.

INFECTIOUS DISEASES

From the earliest mortality follow-up, there has been evidence of excess infectious disease deaths among POWs. Cohen and Cooper (1954) reported mortality rates from tuberculosis that were five times higher than expected, and Nefzger (1970) found a pattern of continued high mortality as a result of tuberculosis persisting in PWP after 20 years. The most recent mortality follow-up by Keehn (1980) showed that although excess tuberculosis mortality in PWP was highest in the years just after repatriation, tuberculosis rates were still roughly twofold higher than expected up to 30 years after repatriation.

Richardson's study of 100 Hong Kong prisoners of the Japanese (1965) found that during 1946–1964, there were 12 deaths from pulmonary tuberculosis whereas only 5 would have been predicted, had the group been dying at rates comparable to those of the Canadian population. In a 1946–1963 mortality follow-up of some 14,000 Australian ex-prisoners of the Japanese, Freed and Stringer (1968) found tuberculosis to be responsible for higher than expected death rates in the later (1951–1963) but not the earlier

(1946–1950) period. A more recent mortality study comparing 908 Australian ex-prisoners with 797 other veterans of the same theater found that mortality differences were pronounced from 5 to 14 years after the war; further analyses, however, did not suggest that these mortality differences could be attributed to particular causes of death (Dent et al., 1989). Moreover, the proportions of subjects whose vital status could not be ascertained differed among POWs (10%) and controls (15%); as a result, the possibility of bias in the study has been raised (Adena, 1989). In a 1973 study comparing samples of New Zealand ex-prisoners (N = 246), ex-servicemen (who went overseas but were not captured, N = 240), and ex-homeservicemen (who did not serve overseas, N = 209), Salmond and colleagues (1977) found a current disablement pension rate for pulmonary tuberculosis of 0% for ex-servicemen, 4.3% for ex-prisoners, and 7.1% for ex-homeservicemen; similar rates for tropical and parasitical disease were 7.1% for ex-servicemen, 1.1% for ex-prisoners, and 0% for ex-homeservicemen.

Turning to morbidity data, in the 1967 follow-up, Beebe (1975) found significantly higher hospitalization rates among PWP, compared with their controls, for pulmonary tuberculosis, early syphilis, amebiasis, schistosomiasis, and other worm infestation; PWK showed significantly higher rates of pulmonary tuberculosis, amebiasis, dysentery, and other worm infestation. A more recent study of 602 former British prisoners of the Japanese, conducted in Liverpool and published by Gill and Bell (1980), found 88 with strongyloidiasis and 6 with intestinal amebiasis. In a study of 170 Australian former prisoners of war of the Japanese and 172 non-POW veteran controls, Goulston et al. (1985) found 6 current cases of strongyloidiasis, all among POWs (for a rate of 3.5%) and all ascertained by microscopy or culture. However, these investigators reported lifetime prevalence rates of 15% for their Australian POWs and 2% for controls, speculating that their low yield of strongyloidiasis was probably the result of less time spent on direct microscopy. Hill (1988), reporting on former British POWs examined at Princess of Wales Royal Air Force Hospital in Ely, stated that the prevalence rate he found, 16%, was perhaps an underestimate and that 20% might be more realistic. The diagnosis of strongyloidiasis may be aided by the recent development of an ELISA test, evaluated in a sample of American POWs by Pelletier et al. (1988).

In the examination study, lifetime prevalence rates of infectious disease were extremely high, from 95% to 100%, for both POWs and controls, but current rates were roughly 20–30% in both POWs and controls, with the exception of WE, who had a low rate of 7.4% (see Table 5.C.3). There were no noteworthy differences between POWs and controls; therefore, no infectious diseases other than dysentery were singled out for further analysis. However, detailed tabulations were produced (see Appendix C), aggregated to the three-digit ICD [International Classification of Diseases] code level, in which each *mention* of an unresolved condition was recorded. Because a particular condition might be mentioned several times in the record of an examination, rates derived from these tabulations are not strictly comparable to the person-based prevalence rates reported elsewhere in this study, nor do they have a straightforward interpretation, given the possibility of multiple mentions of the same condition for a single person.

Nevertheless, these detailed data include only 2 mentions of amebiasis (1 from PWP and 1 from PWK), 10 mentions of dysentery (1 PWP, 2 PWEM, and 7 PWK), and 5 mentions of other helminthiases (all PWP). This latter category included strongyloidiasis, a condition that Gill and Bell (1980) found in nearly 15% of their examinees. Pulmonary tuberculosis was mentioned 16 times (13 PWP and 3 PWK); the most mentioned infectious condition was dermatophytosis: 52 (PWP), 23 (PWEM), 17 (PWE), 118 (PWK), 17 (WP), 0 (WE), and 25 (WK). Dividing these counts by the number of exams gives respective rates of 20.8%, 27.7%, 12.0%, and 28.9% for POWs, and 31.5%, 0%, and 24.3% for controls.

MALIGNANT NEOPLASMS

There was no evidence of increased death rates from malignant neoplasms among POWs in either Nefzger's (1970) or Keehn's (1980) follow-ups, and Beebe (1975) found no significantly greater hospitalization rates for any type of cancer. Although a mortality study of British POWs by Gill (1983), based on death certificates sent in by relatives at the request of national and local POW organizations in the north of England, found higher rates of stomach, pancreas, and liver cancer compared with population values, these findings are clearly vulnerable to selection bias. In a recent study of 908 Australian ex-prisoners and 797 controls, there was no evidence of a higher rate of malignancies among former POWs (Dent et al., 1989). In a 1973 study comparing samples of New Zealand ex-prisoners ($N = 246$), ex-servicemen (who went overseas but were not captured, $N = 240$), and ex-homeservicemen who did not serve overseas ($N = 209$), Salmond and colleagues (1977) found 1.4% of ex-servicemen under current medical supervision for neoplasms versus 0% for both ex-prisoners and ex-homeservicemen.

The examination data also support the contention that military captivity is not associated with increased rates of subsequent malignancy. Lifetime prevalence rates of malignancy are around 15–20% for POWs (except for 9% for PWK); current prevalence rates are 2–5% for all POW groups. None of these rates is appreciably different from its comparable control rate. Lifetime rates of benign neoplasm are approximately the same as malignancy rates, whereas current rates—10–12% for all POWs—are somewhat higher than the malignancy rates. Again, however, there are no noteworthy differences between POWs and controls.

DIABETES

Diabetes mellitus occurs in two distinct forms, insulin-dependent diabetes mellitus (IDDM) and non-insulin-dependent diabetes mellitus (NIDDM). Presumably, the military's medical screening process during admission removes applicants with IDDM, leaving NIDDM as the condition of principal interest in this report. Although the prevalence of diabetes increases with age and other factors can place a person at increased risk of NIDDM, the only factor that has been consistently related to an increased prevalence of diabetes mellitus is higher relative body weight (National Research Council, 1989). Because of this link with body weight, diabetes was singled out from endocrine diseases for special consideration. It is unclear, however, what kind of hypothesis should be formed a priori for POWs, because one might argue either of two ways: earlier starvation lowered the risk of diabetes at the time of captivity and lifetime risks should therefore remain lower, or the recovery from starvation, which might have resulted in an excess weight gain, subsequently raised the lifetime risk of diabetes.

Earlier studies of the MFUA cohort showed that POW death rates for diabetes were substantially below comparable U.S. general population figures (Keehn, 1980), but this finding was true for controls as well and may be attributable to the aforementioned medical screening of military service personnel. Beebe (1975) found no excess hospitalization for diabetes.

Data from the current examination show no evidence for either a higher or lower prevalence of diabetes in POWs. Lifetime prevalence rates for POWs are 12–15% compared with 7–11% for controls (except for a WP rate of 18.5%); current rates are nearly identical to lifetime rates. Diabetes prevalence rates were nonetheless slightly higher among POWs who lost more than 35% of body weight during captivity; they showed no uniform gradient with prison camp symptoms. The simple association with weight loss, however, could have been unduly influenced by differences among POW groups; group-specific correlation analyses showed no evidence of noteworthy correlations. There is, in short, no compelling evidence that diabetes is more or less prevalent among POWs than among controls, based on exam data.

OTHER ENDOCRINE DISEASES

The category of other endocrine diseases includes the nutritional deficiency diseases, for which there is ample evidence of elevated prevalence among POWs. The repatriation examinations of 4,618 PWP by the Morgan Board Debarkation Hospitals (Morgan et al., 1946) produced significant evidence of avitaminosis, with beriberi—resulting from a thiamin (vitamin B_1) deficiency—one of the most prevalent prison camp symptoms; a history suggesting wet beriberi was found in 77% and dry beriberi in 50% of those examined by the Morgan Board. In Beebe's follow-up (1975), significantly higher rates of both beriberi and other avitaminoses among PWP were still found 20 years after repatriation.

The exam data indicated lifetime prevalence rates of other endocrine diseases of between 70–85% among POWs, compared with 50–70% for controls; both PWP and PWK showed appreciably higher rates than their comparable controls. Data from Eberly and Engdahl's (1991) examination study showed lifetime prevalence rates for beriberi of 48% for PWP and 17% for PWK, which are fairly comparable to exam data rates of 61% for PWP and 26% for PWK. There were, however, no noteworthy differences between POWs and controls in current rates of other endocrine diseases, except that PWP had an appreciably lower rate than WP. Thus, appreciably higher rates of other endocrine diseases seen in earlier studies were not seen in the current data. The sequelae of malnutrition and avitaminosis that manifest themselves in other organ systems will be discussed under those systems.

BLOOD DISEASES

Although the repatriation examinations of PWP (Morgan et al., 1946) reported a high rate of anemia (52% of the first 1,500 prisoners surveyed), by the time of Beebe's 1967 study, hospitalization rates of POWs and controls for diseases of the blood and blood-forming organs showed no significant differences (Beebe, 1975). It was therefore somewhat surprising to find appreciably lower lifetime prevalences of blood diseases among PWP and PWK—14% and 12%, respectively—compared with WP and WK—29.6% and 22.3%, respectively (see Table 4.2). Current prevalence rates of blood diseases showed similar and, again, noteworthy differences of 12.4% and 11.5% versus 25.9% and 21.4%, respectively, for PWP and PWK versus WP and WK.

Further analyses of these differences in blood disease prevalence showed that most of this deficit was attributable to lower rates of anemia (ICD codes 280–285). When anemia alone was considered (see Chapter 6), again, there were noteworthy differences in prevalence between PWP and PWK and their respective control groups: 6.8% and 5.2% for PWP and PWK, versus 20.4% and 18.5% for WP and WK. The possibility exists, of course, that it is the control rates that are elevated; however, the corresponding WE rate, 11.1%, although lower than either the WP or WK rate, was nevertheless still higher than the PWP and PWK rates, suggesting that it is the POW rates that are low and not the control rates that are high.

Yet further analyses of the data on the prevalence of anemia shed no additional light on this unanticipated finding; no noteworthy associations were found between anemia prevalence and weight loss or anemia prevalence and symptom score in any of the univariate or multivariate analyses. Even so, the correlation analysis showed small, *negative* correlations between anemia prevalence and both weight loss and prison camp symptoms, indicating that the greater the weight loss and number of prison camp symptoms reported, the *lower* the current prevalence of anemia. Thus, although the finding that anemia is less prevalent among former POWs than among comparable controls appears to be genuine, it is unexplained by simply measured factors such as percent weight loss and the presence of medical symptoms during captivity.

PSYCHIATRIC ILLNESSES (PSYCHOSES AND NEUROSES)

All earlier follow-ups of the MFUA cohort have shown that increased psychiatric illness among POWs was the most striking and persistent aftereffect of military captivity. Cohen and Cooper (1954) found higher death rates for suicide (based on quite small numbers) and for accidental deaths; they also found elevated rates of hospitalization for psychoneurosis in both Pacific and European theater prisoners. Nefzger (1970) found that suicides, although few in number, were about 30% more frequent among Pacific prisoners than among their controls, and Keehn (1980) found later suicide rates to be significantly elevated in PWP but not in the other groups. Such mortality findings, however, are not fully indicative of levels of psychiatric illness, which are more appropriately reflected in morbidity data.

In the 1967 follow-up by Beebe, psychiatric illness was clearly the most prevalent aftereffect of captivity (Beebe, 1975). Compared with controls, PWP, PWE, and PWK groups all showed significantly higher rates of hospitalization for mental, psychoneurotic, and personality disorders. Hospitalization rates for the following specific conditions were significantly higher for POWs than for corresponding controls: schizophrenic disorders (PWP), alcoholic psychoses (PWP), anxiety reaction with somatization (PWP, PWE, and PWK), neurotic-depressive reaction (PWP and PWK), psychoneurosis with somatization (PWP and PWE), other psychoneurotic disorders (PWP), pathological personality (PWP), and alcoholism (PWP). Although all three POW groups showed some elevated hospitalization rates, clearly, the PWP group was most affected.

The 1967 follow-up also included the Cornell Medical Index (CMI), a general health questionnaire with a number of items pertaining to psychological symptoms; when scored in the customary manner, the CMI yields values on several subscales. The scored data showed increased self-reported symptoms for all of the mood and feeling subscales: inadequacy (PWP and PWK), depression (PWP), anxiety (PWP and PWK), sensitivity (PWP and PWK), anger (PWP and PWK), and tension (PWP and PWK), as well as total emotional score (PWP and PWK). The total CMI score (both somatic and psychological) was found to be significantly related to a number of measures of nutritional stress, which are also used in this report for the analyses underlying Table 6.7.

In the latest completed follow-up of the MFUA cohort, which was centered around the Center for Epidemiologic Studies depression (CES-D) scale, Engdahl and Page (1991) found significant and marked elevations in the prevalence of depressive symptoms. In general, rates of depressive symptoms were three to five times higher for POWs than for the general population, and they were positively associated with both weight loss and prison camp symptoms and negatively associated with years of education, age at capture, and being married. (In other words, the more educated, older [when captured], and married POWs were less likely to have depressive symptoms [Page et al., 1991].) Further analysis of the subcomponents of the CES-D showed that these same demographic factors were generally predictive of lower rates of negative affect and higher rates of positive affect, fewer somatic symptoms, and fewer interpersonal problems (Engdahl et al., 1991).

Other recent studies of former American POWs have uncovered similar findings. The results of Eberly and Engdahl (1991) were discussed in an earlier chapter, but it is worth recalling that they showed striking elevations in diagnoses of posttraumatic stress disorder (PTSD) and generalized anxiety among POWs and some elevation of depressive symptoms, even though the Minneapolis depression data were collected using different, and possibly more stringent, diagnostic criteria than were applied in collecting the MFUA data. In an earlier study of 188 former WW II POWs in the Minneapolis area, Kluznick et al. (1986) found a lifetime prevalence of PTSD of 66% and a lifetime prevalence of generalized anxiety disorder of 53%; the prevalence of chronic, unresolved PTSD in this group was 47%. Speed and associates (1989) found that the strongest predictors of PTSD in a smaller group of 62 Minneapolis area POWs were proportion of weight lost and experience of torture during captivity; family history of mental illness and preexisting psychopathology were at best only weakly correlated with persistent PTSD symptoms.

Oboler's report (1987) of 190 consecutive protocol examinations at the Denver VA Medical Center stated that 82% of Pacific prisoners (in all, numbering 50) were found to have psychiatric impairment; 60% suffered from anxiety disorder, 28% from PTSD, and an additional 18% from depressive disorder. Among European prisoners, the corresponding percentages were 60%, 33%, 11%, and 21%; for Korean prisoners (who numbered 15), 73% had psychiatric impairment, 60% had anxiety disorders, and 47% had PTSD. One PWK was diagnosed with dysthymic disorder.

Sutker and Allain (1991) of the New Orleans VA Medical Center have recently reported on Minnesota Multiphasic Personality Inventory (MMPI) profiles of 168 former POWs and 67 controls from WW II and the Korean conflict. Their results confirm previous reports that former POWs have higher scores on the hypochondriasis, depression, and hysteria scales of the MMPI. Sutker and colleagues (1991) reported on a battery of tests administered to 22 Korean prisoners and an equal number of controls drawn from the catchment area of the New Orleans VA Medical Center. They found dramatic differences between the two groups on the MMPI subscales for depression and schizophrenia and a higher Mississippi PTSD score among Korean prisoners. Scores on the Beck depression scale and on state and trait anxiety measures were higher, but not significantly, for POWs. Another study based on a sample of 20 Korean conflict prisoners (Sutker et al., 1990) found PTSD in 18 cases (90%); mood disorders were cited in 75% of cases, anxiety disorder other than PTSD in 45%, and alcohol abuse in 20%.

Goldstein and colleagues (1987) studied 41 Pacific prisoners in the Pittsburgh area and found that half met the full diagnostic criteria for PTSD, with 97% reporting some sleep disturbance. The MMPI profile of the group showed elevations of the hypochondriasis, depression, and hysteria scales, suggesting the presence of a pronounced anxiety state with depressive features. Their findings were similar to those of Sutker et al. (1991) noted above and of Klonoff et al. (1976) noted below. A subsequent study of 10 PWP, all of whom reported sleep disturbances and other PTSD-related findings, showed that 6 of the 10 had no stage 4 sleep and had significantly higher mean ventricular brain ratios, which correlated with the number of awakenings (Peters et al., 1990). Without similar data from normal controls, however, these findings could not be specifically related to PTSD.

Zeiss and Dickman (1989) have reported on a statewide sample of 442 Virginia ex-POWs who responded to a questionnaire mailed from the Roanoke VA Regional Office. The three-page questionnaire requested information on PTSD symptoms and included an abbreviated listing of diagnostic criteria; 44% of those mailed a questionnaire responded. Symptoms of a severity consistent with a diagnosis of PTSD occurred in 56% of respondents (55.7% of PWE and 55.1% of PWP), but in contrast to other studies, most predictor variables—duration of internment, age at capture, current age, and duration of current marriage—were not significantly associated with a diagnosis of PTSD. In fact, only rank at capture showed a significant association, and even more surprising, there was no difference in PTSD prevalence between those with a Pacific and those with a European location of captivity. These findings remain anomalous.

Studies of other than American former prisoners have found similar evidence of psychiatric illness. A 1964–1965 study by Richardson of Canadian WW II prisoners of the Japanese who were captured in Hong Kong reported findings from a study group of 100 former prisoners and a control group of 100 of their brothers (Richardson, 1965). Data on the pension status of all 100 prisoners and controls revealed a higher rate for POWs of compensated neuropsychiatric conditions—28 POWs were receiving compensation versus 3 controls. Psychiatric examinations were conducted on only a smaller group of 20 prisoners and their brothers (Kral et al., 1967). In this smaller group, there was a significantly higher rate of psychiatric complaints among POWs (12 of 20) than among their brothers (2 of 20), and there were significantly higher rates of tension, anxiety, and depression among the POWs. Klonoff et al. (1976), in their study of Canadian WW II prisoners of the Pacific (N = 34) and European (N = 31) theaters, found an MMPI group profile characterized by elevated hysteria and depression scales.

More recently, Tennant et al. (1986a) studied 170 Australian prisoners of the Japanese and 172 veteran controls. They found elevated rates of clinically diagnosed anxiety and depressive disorders among the POWs—although the finding of a difference in the rates of anxiety in the two groups was not statistically significant—but no difference in alcoholism rates. Their questionnaire study similarly showed excess rates of depressive symptoms among POWs (Tennant et al., 1986b). Further analysis of the data on depressive symptoms showed that self-reported nervous illness during the war and depressive illness since the war were independently and significantly associated in both groups with higher rates of depression, as was unemployment among POWs and not being married among controls. Among controls, education had a significant inverse relationship to depression (i.e., higher education and lower depression); the same type of relationship was seen for socioeconomic status among POWs (Dent et al., 1987).

In contrast, a 1973 study by Salmond and colleagues (1977), comparing samples of New Zealand ex-prisoners (N = 246), ex-servicemen who went overseas but were not captured (N = 240), and ex-homeservicemen who did not serve overseas (N = 209), found low and quite comparable rates of nervous disorders currently under medical supervision among the three groups—7.1%, 7.9%, and 5.9%, respectively. Rates of disability, however, showed a different pattern, with 19.4% of ex-prisoners being disabled for other nervous conditions versus 9.5% of ex-servicemen and 0% of ex-homeservicemen.

Gill and Bell's (1981) study of 602 British former Far East POWs who were examined in Liverpool found 209 (34.8%) with significant psychiatric illness; in only 7 cases was this unrelated to the POW experience. Of the 209, 90 had depression, 57 had anxiety neurosis, and 62 had both. In 1981, Patrick and Heaf published a review of this and other British work, as well as worldwide findings. The review also included major results from studies of other, non-POW captives, such as the work by Eitinger (1964) and Strom (1968) on Norwegian concentration camp survivors and Thygesen et al. (1970) on Danish concentration camp survivors.

The preceding brief review of psychiatric findings among POWs merely indicates the depth of available material in the specific area of POW studies; for example, it omits recent research on Vietnam-era POWs and more general review material on the POW experience (e.g., Ursano and Rundell, 1990). There are additional, more tangential areas that could be profitably reviewed as well if space and time permitted. Certainly, the more general study of combat stress and resulting psychiatric disability is especially pertinent to POW studies; indeed, there are clear parallels between the psychological aftereffects of all types of trauma. This point of view is manifested in current arguments about the diagnostic construct of PTSD. This disorder appears for the first time as such in the third edition (1980) of the American Psychiatric Association's Diagnostic and Statistical Manual of mental disorders (known colloquially as DSM-III) but is said to have been known for hundreds of years, although under different names (Trimble, 1985). Clearly, the study of the psychological effects of military captivity could be set in a wider context, but that is not a part of the current report.

The results of the medical examination survey complement those of previous follow-ups and present new material on PTSD, a particular focus of the exam follow-up because it was an expected comorbid or underlying diagnosis associated with the kinds of depressive symptoms seen earlier in the 1984–1985 follow-up. Overall, the most striking psychiatric sequelae seen in the exam are depressive symptoms, PTSD, and generalized anxiety disorder, paralleling the findings of most other studies of former POWs. The exam data provide additional information, however, on the persistence of psychiatric illnesses—for WW II POWs, now as long as 45 years after repatriation. These exam data show that psychiatric illnesses not only persist but that their rates have diminished little over the years. Lifetime prevalence of depressive disorder, for example, was 52%, 36%, 53%, and 56% among PWP, PWE, PWEM, and PWK, respectively; the corresponding rates for current (i.e., unresolved) conditions are 47%, 32%, 51%, and 51%. The data on PTSD are similar, with lifetime rates of 41%, 23%, 28%, and 39% compared with current rates of 40%, 20%, 28%, and 37%. The data for generalized anxiety disorder constitute a third example with lifetime rates of 44%, 47%, 63%, and 59% compared with current rates of 39%, 39%, 55%, and 54%, respectively. In contrast, the structured clinical interview for DSM-III-R (SCID) data show lifetime prevalence levels of PTSD that are about equal to exam levels—but current PTSD rates that are half that size (except for PWK), a finding more in line with those of other studies. Thus, according to physician diagnosis, the rates of psychiatric illness among POWs have decreased only slightly with the passage of time, no matter what their baseline levels, although this observation is not supported by the SCID data. In any case, it is clear that both PWP and PWK rates of psychiatric illness are appreciably higher than rates for PWE. It should be noted that the diagnoses of PTSD, depressive symptoms, and generalized anxiety—in particular, the first two—overlap substantially and that much additional work would be needed to disentangle them. For example, there is a good deal of overlap in the symptoms—and therefore the diagnoses—of PTSD and depressive symptoms. Moreover, it is conceivable that the POW experience causes depression, which in turn causes PTSD symptoms, or vice versa. Such issues are not addressed in this report.

Before leaving the subject of lifetime prevalence of PTSD, depression, and generalized anxiety disorder, it is worthwhile to place the exam results against a more general backdrop to see the extraordinary group that these former POWs constitute. Various disclaimers have been made—based on the low response rates and the very real potential for serious nonresponse bias—about the ability to draw conclusions from the exam data collected. For the three psychiatric conditions listed above, however, the disclaimers are moot. This assertion will be argued using data from the Epidemiologic Catchment Area (ECA) study, sponsored by the National Institute of Mental Health, which surveyed almost 20,000 Americans at five sites across the country. The study yielded some of the most comprehensive data ever collected on psychiatric illness in the U.S. general population.

Consider first the lifetime prevalence of PTSD. Based on ECA data, Helzer et al. (1987) estimated the prevalence of PTSD among men in the general U.S. population at 0.5%. In contrast, the SCID, for example, estimates the prevalence of PTSD in PWP at 33% and in PWK at 41%—rates some 60 to 80 times higher than those found in the national sample. If one were to recalculate the SCID prevalence rates to include all eligible subjects—respondents and nonrespondents alike—and even if one were to count every nonrespondent as never having had PTSD, the revised SCID prevalence would be roughly cut in half among PWP (who had a 50% response rate) and reduced two-and-a-half-fold among PWP (who had roughly a 40% response rate). These revised, "worst-case" estimates are still around 16% for PWP and PWK—and thus 30-fold higher than the national estimate. Although statistical inferences based solely on the sample data are inappropriate, the kind of worst-case analysis presented here shows that despite the sizable problems caused by nonresponse, it is still possible to conclude that PWP and PWK have a significantly higher prevalence of PTSD than the general population.

One can perform similar kinds of calculations for depressive disorders and generalized anxiety disorder. Among men aged 65 and older (comparable to the WW II POW groups), the ECA's estimate of lifetime prevalence of affective disorders (which includes bipolar I and bipolar II disorders, dysthymia, and major depression) is only 1.6%, for men aged 45–64 (closer in age to the Korean conflict group), it is 3.6% (Robins and Regier, 1991). Again, the comparisons to the MFUA estimates are dramatic: physician estimates of lifetime depressive disorders are more than 30 times higher for

PWP and 16 times higher for PWK. Revising the MFUA rates downward in a worst-case scenario still leaves significantly higher prevalence estimates among the MFUA group. Finally, the ECA lifetime prevalence figures for generalized anxiety disorders range from 2.5% to 4.5% for those 65 years of age and older and from 6% to 7% in the age group 45–64. Physician-based prevalence estimates for generalized anxiety disorder were 44% for PWP and 59% for PWK: again, these are quite sizable discrepancies that stand even if worst-case estimates are calculated. Clearly, PTSD, depressive disorder, and generalized anxiety disorder are significantly more prevalent among PWP and PWK than in the general population.

The examination data also provide additional information on the long-term effects of combat, absent captivity, in the follow-up of the WK control group, which consists of men who were lightly wounded and returned to action. The association of combat trauma with psychiatric illness is well established; thus, it is not surprising that the WK group shows almost uniformly higher rates of psychiatric illness than other control groups. Here, the prevalence of psychiatric illness, although somewhat lower in magnitude than in POWs, appears to be as persistent: this pattern is seen for depressive symptoms (28% lifetime versus 22% current), PTSD (12% lifetime versus 11% current), and generalized anxiety (25% lifetime versus 22% current). Again, however, the SCID data tell a different story for PTSD, showing current prevalence rates that are about half the size of lifetime rates. The kind of worst-case analyses made above are not as enlightening in the WK groups, which had only a 15% response rate. Presuming that nonrespondents are free of psychopathology results in worst-case estimates that are reduced six-and-a-half-fold; estimates of this size are too near those of the general population to conclude that the WK group suffers significant psychiatric ill health. Thus, the study results for WK suggest excess psychological problems but do not constitute definitive evidence.

The Structured Clinical Interview data show lifetime rates that are approximately the same as those from the exam but lower current rates; the data from the Mississippi scale are generally a little higher. Again, there are some noteworthy differences between POWs and controls, but these appear to be war-era specific; the current levels of PTSD according to the Mississippi scale are roughly in line with those found either in the SCID or in the exam. The development and use of this instrument among Vietnam veterans may mean that the current standardized scoring and cut-points should be reevaluated for use in WW II and Korean conflict populations. Data from the Hopkins Symptom Check List (SCL-90) suggest that, in addition to the specific conditions noted above, psychiatric symptoms of all sorts are elevated among former POWs, especially among PWK, PWEM, and PWP.

The additional analyses undertaken in Chapter 6 contribute new information to the subject of psychiatric sequelae in former POWs. Both depressive symptoms and PTSD showed noteworthy simple associations with increased weight loss, a finding confirmed by Eberly and Engdahl in their Minneapolis POWs; depressive symptoms, schizophrenia, PTSD, and generalized anxiety all showed noteworthy simple associations with number of prison camp symptoms. In the logistic regression analysis, however, which controlled simultaneously for weight loss, prison camp symptoms, and group differences, depressive disorder showed a noteworthy association only with other symptoms (i.e., not with edema or visual symptoms); PTSD was associated with visual symptoms and with the PWP and PWK groups, generalized anxiety with other symptoms and PWK, and schizophrenia with PWK status. It is worth noting that because weight loss is also a symptom of depression, for example, controlling for it in multivariate analyses may result in a biased estimate of association.

Interpreting these different associations is not at all straightforward. Because all of the prison camp symptom measures also serve as more general measures of harshness of captivity, they may very well be confounded not only with some outcomes (e.g., weight loss and depression) but also with other measures of general and psychological stress, such as beatings and torture. Thus, although the presence of visual symptoms (associated with PTSD) indicates a deficiency of vitamin A, it would be inappropriate, for example, to speculate on a nutritional link between vitamin A deficiency and subsequent PTSD without some biological basis. Similarly, little can be said about the association of other prison camp symptoms with depressive disorder and generalized anxiety. The noteworthy group differences derived from the use of the logistic model, however, are more easily interpreted: both PWP and PWK have higher rates of PTSD than PWE, even after accounting for weight loss and prison camp symptom measures; and generalized anxiety is especially high among PWK, even after accounting for all other factors.

The data on schizophrenia deserve separate discussion. Lifetime prevalence rates for schizophrenia were around 1%, the rate Eberly and Engdahl (1991) quote as a general population estimate, for both PWP and PWE; PWEM and PWK lifetime rates were 2.3% and 3.4%, respectively. Current and lifetime rates differ little. Current schizophrenia in the combined POW group had a noteworthy association with the number of prison camp symptoms (Table 6.4); in addition, there was a noteworthy negative correlation of weight loss and schizophrenia in PWK (Table 6.5), indicating a higher rate of schizophrenia in those who had *less* weight loss. The logistic model, however, found an appreciable association only with PWK status (a 4.4-fold higher risk), indicating a clear link with PWK status but no noteworthy associations with weight loss or prison camp symptoms. Although the data on schizophrenia are quite sparse, it still appears that PWK have a higher prevalence rate and that for PWK alone, less weight loss is associated with a higher prevalence of schizophrenia. This finding argues against nutritional deficiency as a cause of later illness.

In summary, the data show that a number of specific psychiatric conditions occur more frequently among former POWs—in particular, depression, PTSD, and generalized anxiety disorder. The current exam survey data show that POW rates for these conditions are still higher than control rates some four-and-a-half decades after repatriation and that these excesses are found in data collected by examination, structured interview, and questionnaire. The finding of elevated rates of PTSD, a relatively new diagnostic construct, occurs for the first time in this cohort.

In addition to the simple prevalence rate comparisons of POWs and controls, more sophisticated analyses have linked these increased rates with earlier treatment during captivity. Unfortunately, the markers of captivity stress, weight loss and prison camp symptoms, are not only measures of malnutrition but also of general maltreatment. As a result, their noteworthy associations with psychiatric illness do not tell us a great deal about the specific factors underlying subsequent morbidity.

DISEASE OF THE NERVOUS SYSTEM (INCLUDING PERIPHERAL NERVE DISEASE)

Among PWP, the observations of prison camp physicians linked symptoms of peripheral nerve damage to nutritional deficiencies during captivity. Among American prisoners taken at Bataan and Corregidor, Hibbs (1946) reported that everyone in the camp had one form of beriberi or another at some time. He also noted that more than 75% of men in the camp had the predominately sensory disturbances or painful feet characteristic of "dry" beriberi, although less than 2% of the men developed motor paralysis; at the height of the disease, about 40% had 1^+ to 2^+ exaggeration of deep tendon reflexes. A recent analysis of clandestine medical records from two small camps in Japan—those of Maj. William Stewart of the Niigata POW Camp and of Capt. LaMoyne Bleich of the Oeyama POW camp—document the cumulative incidence of various categories of disease to August 1945 (Roland and Shannon, 1991). In Niigata there were 166 neurological disorders among 448 prisoners, a rate of 37%; in Oeyama there were 87 such disorders among 177 prisoners, a rate of 49%.

A report of Canadian prisoners of the Japanese stated that 84% of the repatriates gave a history of neurologic damage during internment; neurologic damage was still evident in 51% of them after they returned to Canada (Crawford and Reid, 1947). The repatriation examinations of some 4,618 former American POWs of WW II reported by Morgan et al. (1946) documented minimal polyneuritis in 568 cases (184 with diminished tendon reflexes and 409 with impairment of sensation) and pronounced polyneuritis in another 29 subjects (16 with diminished tendon reflexes and 22 with impairment of sensation).

Kral and colleagues (1967) examined a group of 20 Canadian former prisoners of the Japanese and 20 of their brothers then living in the Montreal area. They found a significantly higher prevalence of neurological complaints among POWs compared with controls (15 versus 4); their neurological findings included increased rates of superficial hypesthesia, particularly in the lower extremities (12 versus 3), diminished vibration and position sense (8 versus 0), ataxia of the spinal or motor type (9 versus 1), and cranial nerve involvement—sluggish pupillary response and weakness of the facial nerve (6 versus 0). In a 1973 study comparing samples of New Zealand ex-prisoners (N = 246), ex-servicemen who went overseas but were not captured (N = 240), and ex-homeservicemen who did not serve overseas (N = 209), Salmond and colleagues (1977) found a higher rate (5.3%) of central nervous system disorders under current medical supervision among ex-POWs than among ex-servicemen (1.4%).

At Queen Mary's Hospital, Roehampton, some 4,684 British Far East ex-POWs were examined (Gibberd and Simmonds, 1980), and 679 were found to have a neurological condition. Of these, 593 had either optical atrophy or peripheral neuropathy and no other neurological disease. Gill and Bell (1980) reported that 34 of 602 British ex-POWs examined in Liverpool between 1968 and 1978 had evidence of nutritional neuropathy; their subsequent report (Gill and Bell, 1982) of 898 ex-POWs revealed that 5.5% displayed persistent symptomatic neurological disease. A report by Cruickshank (1961), who spent three-and-a-half years in the Changi Military POW Camp on Singapore Island as a medical specialist, provides observations on diet during captivity and its relation to various deficiency syndromes, most of them affecting the nervous system. He noted that neurological features were present in 229 (57%) of the 400 cases suffering from beriberi; among the first 171 such cases, 22% had motor symptoms only, 31% had sensory symptoms only, and 47% had both kinds of symptoms.

Findings of increased neurological problems were still being seen in Beebe's 1967 follow-up of the MFUA study groups. PWP had significantly higher rates of hospital discharges in the broad category of "nervous system, other than central, and sense organs" (Beebe, 1975), and when attention was restricted to 3-digit ICD codes, a significantly higher rate of PWP hospitalizations appeared in the category "other diseases of the peripheral nerves." PWP also had a significantly higher rate of military service-connected compensation for peripheral neuritis.

In more recent studies of American POWs, Eberly and Engdahl (1991) do not mention peripheral neuropathy, probably owing to the lack of suitable data for control rates, but Oboler (1987) found on current examination that 48% (24 of 50) of Pacific WW II prisoners had objective evidence of a persistent peripheral sensory neuropathy. The majority reported only mild symptoms of numbness and tingling, but there were some cases with more severe symptoms, such as "burning" or "electric" sensations that were aggravated by movement and pressure. Among European prisoners, the prevalence of mild peripheral sensory abnormalities was only 5% (6 of 121); among Korean prisoners the prevalence was 7% (1 of 15).

Hong (1986), of the Livermore, California, VA Medical Center, reported the results of neurological examinations and nerve conduction studies on 52 (32 Pacific and 20 European) WW II POWs. Based on the neurological exam, 25 of the PWP and 9 of the PWE were clinically judged to have persistent peripheral neuropathies. All those with a clinical diagnosis had neurological signs of reduced sensation, and about 60% had symmetrically reduced deep tendon reflexes. Electrodiagnostic findings were consistent with distal polyneuropathy of the axonal degeneration type in 28 (88%) of the 32 PWP with a history of beriberi neuritis; in the PWE, however, only 8 (40%) of 20 had electrodiagnostic abnormalities suggesting chronic neuropathies.

In the current MFUA examination survey, lifetime prevalence of disease of the nervous system was appreciably higher in PWP and PWK, compared with their respective controls, as was the current (unresolved) prevalence; indeed, lifetime and current rates changed little—36% compared with 31% for PWP and 25% compared with 21% for PWK. In the analysis of question E in Chapter 5, PWEM were shown to have higher rates of lifetime peripheral nerve disease, which were mostly due to higher rates of mononeuritis of the upper limb and mononeuritis multiplex, mononeuritis of the lower limb, and hereditary and idiopathic peripheral neuropathy.

The analyses of Chapter 6 thus focused specifically on peripheral neuropathy and showed higher rates of current peripheral nerve disease among PWP and PWK. Peripheral neuropathy had a noteworthy association, among all POWs, with both weight loss and prison camp symptoms; in PWP it was appreciably correlated with prison camp symptoms and in PWE, with both weight loss and prison camp symptoms. Logistic regression analysis showed that when prison camp symptoms were redefined into three groups—edema, visual symptoms, and other symptoms—peripheral nerve disease had an appreciable association only with edema: those POWs who reported swelling in the ankles, feet, or legs while in the prison camp had 2.4 times the risk of developing subsequent peripheral nerve disease.

Although all three measures of prison camp symptoms in some part reflect overall harshness of treatment, symptoms of edema have a more specific interpretation. A grossly deficient diet produces protein deficiency and edema, which may be intensified by beriberi heart disease. In addition, the distribution of edema provides important information about its cause:

protein deficiency produces a more generalized edema, whereas edema associated with heart problems tends to be more extensive in the legs (Wilson et al., 1991, p. 232). Thus, self-reported edema in the feet, ankles, and legs is presumably related to beriberi heart disease ("wet" beriberi) in prison camp, which is caused by thiamin deficiency, and that same B_1 deficiency is also the cause of acute peripheral nerve disease ("dry" beriberi). The acute relationship between edema and peripheral nerve disease in prison camp is well established. An appreciable association between edema and chronic peripheral nerve disease, now observed some four-and-a-half decades later, has also been established. However, the pathophysiological processes that might link the two, if there are any, have not yet been established.

Finally, optic nerve disease has been associated with malnutrition in POWs. Bell and O'Neill examined 560 members of the Winnipeg Grenadiers who had been held captive by the Japanese for nearly four years and reported a 20% rate of partial optic atrophy (Bell and O'Neill, 1947). This condition was rarely found, however, during the current exam. As mentioned earlier, detailed tabulations, aggregated to the 3-digit ICD code level, recorded each *mention* during the exam of an unresolved condition. Because a particular condition might be recorded several times in an examination, the rates derived from the detailed tabulations are not strictly comparable to the person-based prevalence rates reported elsewhere. These detailed diagnostic data (see Appendix C) included only 26 mentions of current disorders of the optic nerve (ICD code 377): 9 for PWP, 1 for PWE, and 16 for PWK. Optic nerve disorder was not mentioned in any of the control examinations.

DISEASES OF THE SENSE ORGANS

During the first six years after liberation, Cohen and Cooper (1954) found higher hospitalization rates among PWP than among controls for deafness (3% versus 0.2% in WP), other ear conditions (3% versus 1% in WP), and eye conditions that were not due to nutritional deficiency (3% versus 0.6%). In similar data for PWE there were no differences worth noting. Beebe's 1967 follow-up found significantly higher hospitalization rates among PWP for other diseases of the eye and for otitis media without mastoiditis; among PWK, higher rates were seen for other deafness.

In the current exam survey, lifetime prevalence rates of sense organ disease were quite high among both POWs and controls, generally from 80–90%, with no noteworthy differences seen between the two groups. The prevalence rates for current (unresolved) conditions were nearly identical to the lifetime figures. Given the lack of specific medical hypotheses, no further formal analyses were undertaken.

CARDIOVASCULAR DISEASE (INCLUDING HEART DISEASE, CEREBROVASCULAR DISEASE, HYPERTENSION, AND OTHER CIRCULATORY DISEASES, SUCH AS PERIPHERAL ARTERY DISEASE)

In the first follow-up of the MFUA cohort, Cohen and Cooper (1954) reported that there were 58 PWP deaths in the first six years after liberation, compared with an expected 25.3 deaths (based on U.S. white male mortality rates). Eight of these deaths had cardiovascular disease as an underlying cause; 4.1 such deaths would have been the expected number. However, by the time of Nefzger's follow-up, through 1965, cardiovascular death rates were *below* comparable U.S. general population rates for every POW and control group save PWK. Nefzger (1970) further noted that mortality ratios (calculated by dividing observed by expected deaths) for arteriosclerotic heart disease were slightly larger than those for all vascular disease in the WW II groups, whereas the reverse held true for PWK. This finding suggested that the rate of arteriosclerotic heart disease deaths might have been reduced in the first few years after liberation. Closer inspection of mortality ratios in 4-year intervals, however, offered no support for this hypothesis. All study groups were still too young for cerebrovascular death to have been a frequent cause of death.

Keehn (1980), like Nefzger, found that mortality from cardiovascular disease was below comparable U.S. rates for all six groups of POWs and controls. No relationship between former POW status and level of mortality was apparent, even when an additional 155 deaths mentioning cardiovascular conditions (but not as the underlying cause) were included. Hypertension was mentioned with similar frequency on the death certificates of former POWs and controls.

In Beebe's 1967 morbidity follow-up, hospitalizations for circulatory system disease were significantly higher among PWP compared with controls and, in the early follow-up years, among PWK (Beebe, 1975). Investigations of detailed three-digit ICD codes showed that PWP had rates of arteriosclerotic heart disease and benign essential hypertension that were significantly higher than those of controls.

Gill's (1983) report of mortality and autopsy findings among former British Far East POWs showed a proportion of deaths from ischemic heart disease that was roughly equal to the rate seen in the general population of England and Wales and lower than the rate seen in Scotland. The proportion of deaths that mentioned rheumatic heart disease as the underlying cause was larger among POWs than for these comparison groups, but this amounted to only 6 cases; the proportion of deaths attributable to cerebrovascular disease was roughly the same in ex-POWs as in the general population. Autopsy findings were available for one case with cardiac beriberi, but a further case, although consistent with a diagnosis of chronic cardiac beriberi, could not be confirmed because of the presence of long-standing rheumatic mitral valve disease. Gill states that the difficulty with the last case is fairly common, noting that "the histological changes induced by cardiac beriberi are fairly stereotyped, but are not pathognomic." It should be kept in mind, however, that this study was based on death certificates sent in by relatives at the request of national and local POW organizations in the north of England. The study findings thus are clearly vulnerable to selection bias.

In Richardson's study of 100 Canadian prisoners of the Japanese, which used 100 of their brothers as controls, there was no evidence of increased hypertension; the proportion of POWs with diagnosed hypertension was 15% versus 14% for controls. Atherosclerotic heart disease was present in 3 POWs and 4 controls, and nondiagnostic electrocardiogram data had almost identical rates (12% and 13%). There was, however, a notable difference between former POWs and their brothers in those reporting symptoms of dyspnea on effort without chest pain (28% versus 12%, respectively) and in the reported history of feet sensitive to cold (45% versus 24%, respectively). Thus, Richardson concludes that "the data obtained by clinical examination in this survey do not suggest a significant difference between ex-prisoners and their brothers in the prevalence or severity of cardiovascular disease," adding, however, that "it is possible that significant differences would be found in a larger series" (Richardson, 1965, p. 50).

Richardson found a different story in the Canadian POW mortality data. Using Canadian vital statistics data for the years 1946–1964, he calculated the number of expected deaths that would have been observed in the group had they died at the published Canadian death rates. During this period there were a few more deaths from all causes than expected (135 versus 119.08), but this increase was not statistically significant. In contrast, deaths from atherosclerotic heart disease during the period numbered 47—compared with only 29.94 expected—which was a highly significant excess (p = .01). Richardson notes that the abnormally high atherosclerotic heart disease rate and approximately normal overall death rate are difficult to explain, yet judges that for whatever cause, "it seems necessary to conclude that service in the Far East has probably played some part in the unfavourable mortality experience from atherosclerotic heart disease."

In contrast, a 1973 study by Salmond and colleagues (1977) that compared samples of New Zealand ex-prisoners, ex-servicemen who went overseas, and ex-homeservicemen who did not serve overseas found current disablement pension rates for circulatory system disorders of 4.3%, 0%, and 7.1%, respectively. Gill and Bell's (1981) study of British POWs examined at Liverpool reported that 17% of their series of 602 examinees had ischemic heart disease diagnosed either clinically or by electrocardiography (ECG), and that the overall ECG abnormality rate was 13%. These rates were not thought to be excessive.

Freed and Stringer's (1968) study of mortality among more than 14,000 Australian POWs during 1946–1963 showed an overall significant deficiency of deaths from arteriosclerotic and degenerative heart disease, both during the earlier period (1946–1950) of follow-up—23 observed versus 40.7 expected—and later (1951–1963)—293 observed versus 370.3 expected. Both of these differences were statistically significant. The authors also observed that this deficit was most marked in the older age groups. A recent mortality study of 908 Australian ex-POWs and 797 other veterans found a higher proportion of deaths from ischemic heart disease among POWs but a lower proportion of ischemic heart disease, other heart disease, and cerebrovascular disease. None of these differences, however, was exceptional, and overall, the cause of death was not associated with POW status. This study relied on other than official records; because the proportions of subjects whose vital status could not be ascertained differed among POWs (10%) and controls (15%), the possibility of bias has been raised by other researchers (Adena, 1989).

Recent morbidity data on cardiovascular disease in former POWs come from the Eberly and Engdahl and the Oboler studies. As Chapter 4 noted, Eberly and Engdahl (1991) found lower than expected lifetime prevalence rates of hypertension, cerebrovascular accident, myocardial infarction, and intermittent claudication among Minneapolis POWs, compared with general population rates. However, the rates in the Minneapolis group for conditions other than hypertension were also lower than examination rates in the MFUA study for both POWs and controls, raising the possibility that the Minneapolis POW group was healthier than the MFUA's national sample. Recent data collected by Oboler (1987) at the Denver VA Medical Center report the occurrence of hypertension in 34% of PWP, 33% of PWE, and 27% of PWK; these figures are a little lower than those of Eberly and Engdahl but still roughly comparable to the MFUA rates. Oboler reports no findings consistent with chronic beriberi heart disease and states that "no definite connection could be drawn between these veterans' POW confinement and their current cardiovascular disease."

The examination data showed no appreciably higher lifetime prevalence rates among POWs for either heart disease, cerebrovascular disease, or hypertension and other circulatory diseases (Table 4.2), nor were there any differences in current prevalence rates (Table 5.C.3). In Chapter 6, however, the analysis focused on more narrowly defined medical conditions. Although there were no noteworthy differences between POWs and controls in the prevalence of hypertension, cerebrovascular disease, or myocardial infarction, PWEM showed an appreciably higher rate of ischemic heart disease than did WE—28% compared with 7%. Further analyses showed no noteworthy associations with either weight loss or prison camp symptoms, but the Cochran-Mantel-Haenszel analysis found an appreciable association of ischemic heart disease with prison camp symptoms, after controlling for POW group differences.

Logistic model analyses showed the prevalence of ischemic heart disease to be 1.7 times higher among POWs who reported edema in prison camp than in POWs who did not report it—a new finding; they also demonstrated that ischemic heart disease was, in addition, only about half as prevalent among PWK, probably owing to their younger age. The prevalence of cerebrovascular disease was possibly associated with the number of visual symptoms (persistent difficulty seeing in the dark, etc.), each additional symptom increasing the risk of cerebrovascular disease 1.7 times—again, a new finding among POWs.

Although the appreciable association between increased prevalence of ischemic heart disease later in life among POWs and self-reported symptoms of edema in prison camp is new, the acute cardiac effects of nutritional deprivation are well known. Unlike the situation for psychiatric conditions, the reporting of edema in prison camp is not only a general measure of stress but also indicates a specific nutritional deficiency, beriberi. A grossly deficient diet produces protein deficiency and edema, which may be intensified by beriberi heart disease. As noted earlier, the distribution of edema provides important information about its cause, with protein deficiency producing a more generalized edema and heart disease producing an edema that tends to be more extensive in the legs (Wilson et al., 1991, p. 232). Thus, the self-reported edema in the feet, ankles, and legs is presumably related to beriberi heart disease ("wet" beriberi) in prison camp, which is caused by thiamin deficiency. There have been difficulties in linking beriberi with subsequent heart disease in clinical studies because typical medical findings are consistent with beriberi heart disease but are not pathognomic (recall Gill above). The examination data from the current study now provide epidemiologic evidence to suggest that earlier treatment in prison camp is linked to increased ischemic heart disease four-and-a-half decades later. However, one must interpret this association cautiously because it has no established pathophysiologic basis.

The increased prevalence of cerebrovascular disease among POWs that is associated with increased reporting of visual symptoms appears to be an entirely new finding without strong accompanying clinical evidence. Visual symptoms, like edema, are thought to be fairly specific evidence of nutritional deficiency, in this case vitamin A. Although vitamin A is necessary to maintain epithelial tissue and there has been great interest in the inverse association of vitamin A and cancer, a potential link between earlier vitamin A deficiency and subsequent excess stroke 45 years later must be considered highly speculative.

Peripheral arterial disease (PAD), whose assessment typically includes a history of intermittent claudication, deserves separate mention. Intermittent claudication was seen at such an appreciably higher level in the MFUA sample than in the Eberly and Engdahl (1991) sample that it might have been dismissed as an artifact of the exam process, especially since there were no appreciable differences between lifetime prevalences for MFUA POWs and controls. Instead, the analyses of Chapter 6, discussed below, linked PAD to earlier treatment in prison camp.

There are few systematic prevalence data on PAD in populations, an exception being the Criqui et al. (1985) population-based study of a sample of whites averaging 66 years of age. The study showed that large-vessel PAD was present in 12% of that group, which was within the range of the examination findings. In general, however, PAD is characteristically a disease of old age, and its risk factors are similar to those for cardiovascular heart disease and stroke—cigarette smoking, diabetes, systolic blood pressure, and serum cholesterol (Fowkes et al., 1992). Unfortunately, data on PAD risk factors such as smoking and cholesterol were not routinely collected in the examination.

In the exam data, the current prevalence of intermittent claudication and of arterial vascular disease had separate, noteworthy associations with percent weight loss and number of prison camp symptoms. The logistic regression analysis, however, showed that for both conditions the only noteworthy association was with weight loss, with each additional 10% of precaptivity weight loss increasing the prevalence of disease by 30–40%. The lack of association with symptoms indicating a specific deficiency, such as in the case of ischemic heart disease and cerebrovascular disease, combined with little clinical information on nutritional risk factors, makes further explication of this finding impossible.

ACUTE AND CHRONIC RESPIRATORY DISEASE

For the six years following liberation, Cohen and Cooper (1954) reported higher hospitalization rates for PWP compared with controls for respiratory diseases other than pneumonia—17% for PWP versus 5% in controls; Beebe (1975) also reported higher rates for PWP and for PWE in the broad rubric of respiratory conditions. However, there were no significant differences between POWs and controls in any of the detailed three-digit diagnostic data.

Gill and Bell (1981) note that no other surveys have sought data on the prevalence of respiratory disease in former Far East POWs and cite a rate of chronic bronchitis of 22% (135 of 602 former POWs examined in Liverpool); this rate is thought to be about double that of the comparable general population. They investigated respiratory disease further by reviewing chest x rays and comparing them with a randomly chosen group of controls, matched on age, sex, and social class. These efforts produced radiologic evidence of significantly more thickened pleura, old rib fractures, emphysema, and diffuse fibrosis among the POWs. Unfortunately, Gill and Bell had no data on smoking, but they noted that recurrent attacks of bronchitis were common in captivity. They also noted that work in dusty environments was common among POWs, which could have relevance for their findings of excess diffuse pulmonary fibrosis. In Gill's study of mortality and autopsy findings (Gill, 1983), however, the proportion of deaths from chronic bronchitis was nearly identical in former POWs and in the general population of Scotland; it was smaller in POWs than in the general population of England and Wales. Dent et al. (1989) likewise show a smaller proportion of deaths resulting from respiratory disease in POWs than in comparable controls.

Compared with controls, the examination data show an appreciably higher lifetime prevalence of acute respiratory disease among PWK only and no noteworthy differences for chronic disease. For current (unresolved) respiratory disease, there were no noteworthy differences between POWs and controls for either acute or chronic conditions. In Chapter 6, asthma was specifically selected for further study, based on clinical judgment, but, again, there were no appreciable differences in prevalence between POWs and controls. Analyses of the relationship of asthma and prison camp treatment, however, revealed a noteworthy association of asthma with prison camp symptoms, and in PWP the current prevalence of asthma was appreciably correlated with both weight loss and prison camp symptoms.

In the logistic regression analysis, an increased prevalence of asthma was associated with increased visual symptoms, and each additional reported symptom increased the prevalence by roughly 29%. Other factors being equal, PWK had about half the prevalence of WW II POWs, a finding that is probably related to age. The noteworthy association of asthma with visual symptoms (similar to that seen for stroke) raises again the intriguing possibility that the observed excess prevalence of asthma might be nutritionally related, because the reporting of visual symptoms is fairly specific evidence of vitamin A deficiency and vitamin A is necessary for the maintenance of epithelial tissue. Again, however, there is little other evidence for such an association, and any hypothesis linking vitamin A deprivation and subsequent asthma (45 years later) must be considered highly speculative.

DIGESTIVE DISEASES

During the first six years following repatriation, Cohen and Cooper (1954) reported higher rates of hospitalization for gastritis, enteritis, and functional intestinal disorders among PWP (6%) and PWE (5%), compared with controls (1% and 0.2%, respectively). Beebe (1975) found increased hospitalization rates among PWP for "gastroenteritis and colitis, except ulcerative," and for "other diseases of the intestines and peritoneum." He further stated that VA compensation data suggested an excess of peptic ulcer, both for PWP (with a compensation rate of 4.2% versus 0.6% for WP) and for PWK (4.0% versus 0.7% for WK).

Richardson's (1965) study of 100 former Canadian prisoners and an equal number of their brothers showed an increased history of liver disease in POWs (25 versus 13) and of nonspecific gastrointestinal symptoms with no diagnosis (47 versus 34). A relatively high incidence of irritable bowel syndrome was also noted. Special attention was paid to the diagnosis of peptic ulcer, with the finding that 21 POWs had such a diagnosis (current or during 1946–1964) compared with 8 controls; 11 POWs had been granted a pension for their ulcers compared with 2 controls. The locations of these ulcers were gastric (4 POWs, 2 controls), duodenal (13 POWs, 5 controls), and unspecified (4 POWs, 1 control). Within the past two years, 17 POWs had had symptoms versus only 5 controls. A review of records for all ex-prisoners living in Canada found a prevalence rate of 15.7% for peptic ulcer.

In a 1973 study comparing samples of New Zealand ex-prisoners, ex-servicemen who went overseas, and ex-homeservicemen who did not serve overseas, Salmond and colleagues (1977) found rates of digestive system disorders under current medical supervision of 12.4%, 8.6%, and 7.4%, respectively. Rates for disablement pensions, however, were nearly equal: 7.5%, 7.1%, and 7.1%. Ex-prisoners had a higher rate of current stomach trouble (36.1%) than did ex-servicemen (23.5%) or ex-homeservicemen (14.8%). Eighty percent of those with present symptoms of stomach trouble also had such symptoms at the time of their discharge from the service.

Goulston et al. (1985) studied gastrointestinal morbidity among 170 former Australian prisoners and 172 comparable controls. They reported that duodenal ulcers were significantly more prevalent among former POWs (24.7%) than among controls (10.5%), a finding that was confirmed by the observation that a higher proportion of POWs were taking cimetidine (9.0%) compared with controls (2.3%). They reported no other significant differences between the two groups in gastrointestinal disease.

Gill and Bell (1981) performed single-contrast barium meal examinations of all Far East POWs examined at Liverpool during 1968–1978 who complained of significant dyspepsia. They found evidence of duodenal ulceration in 48 patients, out of a total of 602 POWS examined, for a rate of 8.0%; an additional 6.8% had been successfully treated for duodenal ulcer in the past. These figures were thought to be high, compared with an earlier British estimate.

The examination data showed an appreciably higher lifetime prevalence of digestive disorders among PWK (Table 4.2) than among controls and appreciably higher current prevalences for both PWP and PWK (Table 5.C.3). Comparison of PWEM and PWE lifetime prevalence data showed that gastroenteritis was appreciably more prevalent among PWEM (43%) than among PWE (28%). The analyses of Chapter 6 showed an appreciably higher prevalence of ulcer in PWK and of gastroenteritis in both PWEM and PWK, compared with controls; among all POWs combined, however, neither condition was appreciably associated with either weight loss or prison camp symptoms, nor were there any noteworthy correlations in the individual POW groups.

The logistic regression analysis, however, showed a noteworthy association of ulcer with both visual symptoms and with PWK status, and gastroenteritis had a noteworthy association with the reporting of other symptoms. Each additional reported visual symptom was estimated to increase the current prevalence of ulcer by 15%; all other things being equal, PWK had about 1.8 times as high a prevalence as the WW II POWs. As noted earlier for stroke and asthma, the reporting of visual symptoms is thought to be fairly specific evidence of vitamin A deficiency (vitamin A is necessary for the maintenance of epithelial tissue). Again, however, there is little other evidence for such an association, and any hypothesis linking vitamin A deprivation directly to subsequent ulcer 45 years later must be considered highly speculative. Likewise, there is no specific explanation for the noteworthy association of other symptoms and gastroenteritis, except that the "other symptom" category included reports of prison camp dysentery.

UROGENITAL DISEASES

Cohen and Cooper (1954) reported higher rates of hospitalization in the first six years after repatriation for non-VD genitourinary diseases among PWP (6.5%) compared with WP (1%), but not in PWE (2%) compared with WE (3%). Beebe (1975) observed significantly higher hospitalization rates for genitourinary system disease in PWP than in controls, and, at the three-digit ICD level, significantly higher PWP rates of hospitalization for kidney infections and calculi of the kidney and ureter. Higher rates of genitourinary conditions among POWs have not been cited in the earlier reports of studies on British, Canadian, and Australian POWs, and Salmond et al. (1977) report a lower rate of hospitalization for New Zealand ex-prisoners (6.8%) than for ex-servicemen (8.2%).

The examination data showed an appreciably higher lifetime prevalence of urogenital conditions for PWE compared with WE (Table 4.2), but this is due to a low WE rate rather than a high PWE rate. There were no noteworthy differences in the current prevalence of urogenital conditions (Table 5.C.3). Given the lack of differences and no clear a priori hypotheses, no further analyses were undertaken.

SKIN DISEASE

Diseases of the skin resulted in more frequent hospitalizations for PWP than for WP in the six years following liberation—13% versus 3%—but not for PWE compared with WE—5% versus 4% (Cohen and Cooper, 1954), a finding that was later confirmed by Beebe (1975). Among the detailed diagnoses reported by Beebe, only the PWP hospitalization rates for boil and carbuncle were significantly elevated. Gill and Bell's (1980) report of persisting tropical diseases among former British POWs notes a high prevalence of "creeping eruption" skin rash (a result of infection with *Strongyloidiasis stercoralis* and thus discussed earlier under infectious diseases), of tropical ulcers, and, in one case, of spontaneously occurring keloid scar tissue. There is, however, little or no other mention of skin disease in the published reports cited earlier on Canadian and Australian ex-POWs; moreover, Salmond et al. (1977) report a rate of hospitalization for skin disorders that is lower for ex-prisoners (2.4%) than for ex-servicemen (3.4%).

The examination data showed no appreciably higher lifetime or current prevalence rates of skin conditions among POWs compared with controls (Tables 4.2 and 5.C.3). In the absence of specific hypotheses, no further analyses were undertaken.

ARTHRITIS AND OTHER MUSCULOSKELETAL DISEASES

The rate of hospitalization for diseases of bones and organs of movement was elevated among PWP (8.5%) compared with WP (2%) and somewhat elevated among PWE (3%) compared with WE (1.5%) (Cohen and Cooper, 1954); only PWP showed a significant excess in Beebe's follow-up (1975). The only detailed condition in this broad rubric with a significantly higher PWP hospitalization rate was osteoarthritis and allied conditions.

Richardson (1965) reports on the results of an x ray and clinical survey of disabilities of the cervical and lumbar spine among 96 Canadian prisoners of the Japanese and 96 of their brothers chosen as controls. The radiologic findings showed no appreciable difference between POWs and controls in osteoporosis, disk space narrowing, or osteophyte formation. There were, however, more reported neck and back troubles among the ex-prisoners, and this finding of more frequent symptomatic problems unaccompanied by radiologic evidence could not be satisfactorily explained. Because the study did not establish a statistically significant difference, Richardson concludes: "On the evidence available it is impossible to determine to what extent service-related factors account for this trend."

In a 1973 study comparing samples of New Zealand ex-prisoners, ex-servicemen who went overseas, and ex-homeservicemen who did not serve overseas, Salmond and colleagues (1977) found rates of bone and muscle disorders under current medical supervision of 20.1%, 12.1%, and 8.1%, respectively. Rates of current disablement pensions, however, showed a much different pattern: 18.2% for ex-POWs, 11.9% for ex-servicemen, and 42.9% for ex-homeservicemen. Arthritis or back trouble was reported by 55.1% of ex-POWs, 47.2% of ex-servicemen, and 40.8% of ex-homeservicemen. At the time of their discharge from service, 69% of ex-POWs had such symptoms compared with 38% of ex-servicemen and 35% of ex-homeservicemen.

Oboler's (1987) recent report on ex-POWs examined in the Denver VA Medical Center showed a high prevalence of spinal arthritis in both European and Pacific prisoners; in the European group especially, this condition was related to parachuting from or landing with a disabled aircraft. In the European group, 52% (63 of 121 ex-POWs) had radiographic evidence of spinal arthritis, and 24% had evidence of degenerative arthritis that could be related to the effects of POW capture or captivity. Among Pacific prisoners, 68% (34 of 68) had current evidence of spinal osteoarthritis, with 46% having disease related to earlier POW confinement.

In the examination data, the lifetime prevalence of musculoskeletal disorders among POWs was quite high—87% to 94%; it was appreciably higher among PWK than WK (Table 4.2). Current prevalence rates (Table 5.C.3) of musculoskeletal conditions, however, were nearly the same as lifetime rates, and there were no noteworthy differences between POWs and controls. In Chapter 6, attention was narrowed to osteoarthritis and traumatic arthritis, but, again, there were no noteworthy differences in current prevalence rates (Table 6.1).

Osteoarthritis, however, showed a noteworthy association with weight loss in the group of combined POWs: it was present in 35% of POWs who reported a weight loss of 35% or less and in only 28% of POWs reporting a weight loss of more than 35%. This negative association of weight loss and osteoarthritis—*more* arthritis in those with *less* weight loss—was the only negative association observed among the conditions in Table 6.3; it was also seen in negative correlations between weight loss and osteoarthritis for both PWP and PWK in Table 6.5. Controlling for POW group, there was still some association of osteoarthritis with weight loss.

The logistic regression analysis confirmed these earlier indications, showing that the relative odds of having osteoarthritis (0.88) are smaller by about 12% for every additional 10% of body weight loss during captivity. As noted previously, the effects of additional weight loss are cumulative, and POWs who lost 40% of body weight, for example, have only 60% of the estimated prevalence of osteoarthritis of POWs who reported a weight loss of less than 10%.

This unusual finding was entirely unanticipated and difficult to explain. The data argue against its being a simple statistical artifact because the prevalence of *traumatic* arthritis was *higher* in the high-weight-loss group, no doubt because weight loss was serving as a proxy for general harshness of treatment. Traumatic arthritis also showed small, but positive, correlations with weight loss and with prison camp symptoms, as expected. Thus, osteoarthritis, a clinical condition distinct from traumatic arthritis, showed a disparate pattern of association. The explanation for this finding remains unclear.

CONGENITAL CONDITIONS, SYMPTOMS AND ILL-DEFINED CONDITIONS, INJURY AND POISONING, AND FACTORS INFLUENCING HEALTH STATUS AND CONTACT WITH HEALTH SERVICES (V-CODES)

The medical conditions under these headings have been grouped together because they are all somewhat atypical. Congenital conditions should appear infrequently, if at all, because the military's medical entrance exam is meant to screen out disqualifying, preexisting conditions. Both symptoms and ill-defined conditions, as well as V-codes (i.e., factors influencing health status and contact with health services), are categories containing conditions that did not warrant full, detailed diagnostic coding. Medical conditions that are coded to the injury and poisoning category are likewise unusual because although the injury itself is assigned a code in this category (e.g., fracture of vertebral column), its sequelae are specified under another diagnostic rubric (e.g., traumatic arthritis). These conditions do, nevertheless, indicate an increased burden of illness, however ill defined.

Cohen and Cooper (1954) report appreciably higher hospitalization rates for wounds or injuries, including residual effects and their treatment, in both PWP (20%) and PWE (16%), compared with their respective control groups, WP (4%) and WE (5%). Beebe (1975) reported significantly higher hospitalization rates, compared with controls, for symptoms, for observation and examination only (corresponding most closely to the ICD-9-CM category of V-codes), and for "accidents, poisoning and violence" among PWP and PWK; an increased rate of hospitalization for accidents, poisoning, and violence was seen as well among PWE. There were no significant differences between POWs and controls for hospitalizations for congenital conditions.

Detailed diagnoses associated with POW status in Beebe's follow-up included upper gastrointestinal (GI) symptoms (PWP and PWE), abdominal and lower GI symptoms (PWP), symptoms referable to limbs and back (PWK), nervousness and debility (PWP and PWE), observation without medical care (PWP and PWK), and follow-up examination without medical care (PWP and PWK). Other diagnoses with statistically significant elevations among POWs were fracture of the femur (other than neck) (PWK), multiple open wounds of the face and other sites (PWK), and effects of reduced temperature (PWK). Salmond et al. (1977) report a higher rate of hospitalization for wounds and accidents in New Zealand ex-prisoners (9.6%) than in ex-servicemen (6.8%), but ex-homeservicemen also had a high rate (9.3%). Rates of ill-defined and miscellaneous conditions were 3.4% for ex-servicemen, 2.0% for ex-prisoners, and 4.0% for ex-homeservicemen.

The exam data show low lifetime and current prevalence rates for congenital conditions, with no appreciable differences between POWs and controls—a somewhat reassuring finding. Lifetime and current rates of symptoms and ill-defined conditions are all quite high—97% or more in all but one group—and the only noteworthy difference is between PWK (lifetime rate of 99.3%) and WK (lifetime rate of 94.2%). Lifetime injury and poisoning rates are likewise high, although generally only in the low 90% range, and both PWE and PWEM rates are appreciably higher than the WE rate; here it may be more a reduced WE than increased PWE and PWEM rates that account for this difference. Current rates for injury and poisoning showed no appreciable differences between POWs and controls. Lifetime prevalence rates of V-codes were around 50% in all groups; there were no noteworthy differences. PWP had an appreciably *lower* prevalence of current V-code conditions than did WP, and there were no other noteworthy differences. The ill-defined nature of these findings and their presumed overlap with other, better defined medical conditions argue against further detailed analyses of these results.

SUMMARY

In many instances, the organ-specific findings from this study based on medical examination data are familiar. The appreciably increased prevalence of depressive disorder, PTSD, and generalized anxiety, for example, is not unexpected. Similar findings regarding peripheral nerve disease, ulcer, and gastroenteritis are, likewise, not surprising. Even in these cases, however, there are some intriguing new data on a potential link with nutritional deficiencies, such as between ulcer and earlier visual symptoms (indicating vitamin A deficiency). The noteworthy association between current peripheral nerve disease and earlier edema, itself indicative of a previous vitamin B_1 deficiency, suggests that along with the well-known short-term neurological effects of (dry) beriberi, there may be persistent neurological effects decades after the original nutritional disease has been successfully treated and acute symptoms have abated.

The finding of an increased prevalence of schizophrenia among PWK is new, and an appreciable correlation with weight loss in this group offers further material for speculation. Because schizophrenia has not been linked with psychological trauma, the material basis for the observed association (e.g., an organic brain syndrome associated with injury or nutritional deprivation) could well be something other than general ill treatment; the association may also be a statistical artifact. Findings of increased asthma and cerebrovascular disease in POWs who reported visual symptoms in prison camp are likewise new, and somewhat unexpected. Again, this is an instance of the identification of aftereffects of military captivity accompanied by evidence of a deficiency of vitamin A in prison camp. The findings concerning both intermittent claudication and arterial vascular disease appear for the first time in this cohort, and their associations with percent weight loss do not contribute much to an explanation. The last new finding, an appreciably lower prevalence of osteoarthritis in POWs who reported greater weight loss, is not only unanticipated but in the opposite direction of all the other findings in Chapter 6. No explanations for it come readily to mind.

Last, but certainly not least, is the finding of a noteworthy association between ischemic heart disease and earlier reporting of localized edema. Although there has been much interest in heart disease among former POWs, this result was not entirely expected, given the lack of noteworthy differences between POWs and controls and the fact that other studies have found conflicting evidence from both POW morbidity and mortality data. The lack of a clear biological mechanism linking nutritional deprivation and subsequent *chronic* heart disease requires that one remain somewhat skeptical of this finding of association, especially given the caveats noted earlier in this report regarding the low response rates. Nevertheless, localized edema is a noteworthy risk factor for only two current medical conditions in these POW examinations—peripheral nerve disease and ischemic heart disease—both of which are acutely related to thiamin deficiency, either the "dry" form of beriberi (peripheral nerve disease) or the "wet" form (cardiac problems). The specificity of association between localized edema and the only two medical conditions with well-established acute relationships to thiamin deficiency suggests that the association between earlier nutritional deprivation in prison camp and chronic ischemic heart disease is not an artifact.

Richardson (1965, p. 61) wrote in his earlier report that "the request for progressive increases [in pension] with advancing age would be more impressive if there were evidence of widespread or almost universal deterioration in the health of these veterans with the passing years. There is no evidence that this is the case, although there is evidence that as in any aging population there is an increasing number with serious disability." Excepting psychiatric illness, this report has shown little evidence of widespread ill health among former prisoners of war; even so, the number of specific medical conditions now posited as aftereffects of military captivity continues to grow.

REFERENCES

Adena MA. 1989. The health of Australian veterans. Med. J. Austral. 150:356-357.

Beebe GW. 1975. Follow-up studies of World War II and Korean war prisoners: II. Morbidity, disability, and maladjustments. Am. J. Epidemiol. 101:400-422.

Bell PG, O'Neill JC. 1947. Optic atrophy in Hong Kong prisoners of war. Can. Med. Assoc. J. 56:475-481.

Cohen BM, Cooper MZ. 1954. A Follow-up Study of World War II Prisoners of War. Veterans Administration Medical Monograph. Government Printing Office, Washington, DC.

Crawford JN, Reid JAG. 1947. Nutritional disease affecting Canadian troops held prisoner of war by the Japanese. Can. J. Res. 25(E):53-85.

Criqui MH, Fronek A, Barrett-Connor E, et al. 1985. The prevalence of peripheral arterial disease in a defined population. Circulation 71:510-515.

Cruickshank EK. 1961. Neuro-psychiatric disorders in prisoners-of-war. In Psychiatrie der Gegenwart, Band III. Springer-Verlag, pp. 807-836.

Dent OF, Tennant CC, Goulston KJ. 1987. Precursors of depression in World War II veterans 40 years after the war. J. Nerv. Ment. Dis. 175:486-490.

Dent OF, Richardson B, Wilson S, et al. 1989. Postwar mortality among Australian World War II prisoners of the Japanese. Med. J. Aust. 150:378-382.

Eberly RE, Engdahl BE. 1991. Prevalence of somatic and psychiatric disorders among former prisoners of war. Hosp. Commun. Psychiatry 42:807-813.

Eitinger L. 1964. Concentration Camp Survivors in Norway and Israel. Oslo University Press, Oslo; Allen and Unvin, London.

Engdahl BE, Page WF. 1991. Psychological effects of captivity. In Page WF (ed.), Epidemiology in Military and Veteran Populations, National Academy Press, Washington, DC, pp. 49-66.

Engdahl BE, Page WF, Miller TW. 1991. Age, education, maltreatment, and social support as predictors of chronic depression in former prisoners of war. Soc. Psychiatry Psychiatr. Epidemiol. 26:63-67.

Fowkes FGR, Housley E, Riemersma RA, et al. 1992. Smoking, lipids, glucose intolerance, and blood pressure as risk factors for peripheral atherosclerosis compared with ischemic heart disease in the Edinburgh artery study. Am. J. Epidemiol. 135:331-340.

Freed G, Stringer PB. 1968. Comparative mortality experience, 1946–1963, among former Australian prisoners of war of the Japanese. Aust. Repat. Dept. Med. Bull. 2:28.

Gibberd FB, Simmonds JP. 1980. Neurological disease in ex-Far-East prisoners of war. Lancet ii:135-137.

Gill G. 1983. Study of mortality and autopsy findings amongst former prisoners of the Japanese. J. R. Army Med. Corps 129:11-13.

Gill GV, Bell DR. 1980. Persisting tropical diseases amongst former prisoners of war of the Japanese. Practitioner 224.801-803.

Gill GV, Bell DR. 1981. The health of former prisoners of war of the Japanese. Practitioner 225:531-538.

Gill GV, Bell DR. 1982. Persisting nutritional neuropathy amongst former war prisoners. J. Neurol. Neurosurg. Psychiatry 45:861-865.

Goldstein G, van Kammen W, Shelly C, et al. 1987. Survivors of imprisonment in the Pacific theater during World War II. Am. J. Psychiatry 144:1210-1213.

Goulston KJ, Dent OF, Chapuis PH, et al. 1985. Gastrointestinal morbidity among World War II prisoners of war: 40 years on. Med. J. Aust. 143:6-10.

Helzer JE, Robins LN, McEvoy L. 1987. Post-traumatic stress disorder in the general population. N. Engl. J. Med. 317:1630-1634.

Hibbs RE. 1946. Beriberi in Japanese prison camp. Ann. Intern. Med. 25(2):270-282.

Hill JA. 1988. Strongyloidiasis in ex-Far East prisoners of war (letter). Br. Med. J. 296:753.

Hong CZ. 1986. Electrodiagnostic findings of persisting polyneuropathies due to previous nutritional deficiency in former prisoners of war. Electromyogr. Clin. Neurophysiol. 26:351-363.

Keehn RJ. 1980. Follow-up studies of World War II and Korean war prisoners. III. Mortality to January 1, 1976. Am. J. Epidemiol. 111:194-211.

Klonoff H, Clark C, Horgan J, et al. 1976. The MMPI profile of prisoners of war. J. Clin. Psychol. 32:623-627.

Kluznik JC, Speed N, Van Valkenburg C, Magraw R. 1986. Forty-year follow-up of United States prisoners of war. Am. J. Psychiatry 143:1443-1445.

Kral VA, Pazder LH, Wigdor BT. 1967. Long-term effects of a prolonged stress experience. Can. Psychiatr. Assoc. J. 12:175-181.

Morgan HJ, Wright IS, van Ravensworth A. 1946. Health of repatriated prisoners of war from the Far East. J. Am. Med. Assoc. 130(15):995-999.

National Research Council. 1989. Diet and Health: Implications for Reducing Chronic Disease Risk. National Academy Press, Washington, DC.

Nefzger MD. 1970. Follow-up studies of World War II and Korean war prisoners. I. Study plan and mortality findings. Am. J. Epidemiol. 91:123-138.

Oboler S. 1987. American prisoners of war—an overview. In Williams T (ed.), Post-Traumatic Stress Disorders: A Handbook for Clinicians. Disabled American Veterans, Cincinnati, Ohio, pp. 131-143.

Page WF, Engdahl BE, Eberly RE. 1991. Prevalence and correlates of depressive symptoms among former prisoners of war. J. Nerv. Ment. Dis. 179:670-677.

Patrick DL, Heaf PJD. 1981. Long-term Effects of War-Related Deprivation on Health: A Report on the Evidence. British Members Council of the World Veterans' Federation, London.

Pelletier LL, Baker CB, Gam AA, et al. 1988. Diagnosis and evaluation of treatment of chronic strongyloidiasis in ex-prisoners of war. J. Infect. Dis. 157:573-576.

Peters J, van Kammen DP, van Kammen WB, Neylan T. 1990. Sleep disturbances and computerized axial tomographic scan findings in former prisoners of war. Compr. Psychiatry 31:535-539.

Richardson HJ. 1965. Report of a study of disabilities and problems of Hong Kong veterans, 1964-1965. Canadian Pensions Commission, Ottawa.

Robins LN, Regier DA (eds.). 1991. Psychiatric Disorders in America: The Epidemiologic Catchment Area Study. Free Press, New York.

Roland CG, Shannon HS. 1991. Patterns of disease among World War II prisoners of the Japanese: hunger, weight loss, and deficiency diseases in two camps. J. Hist. Med. Allied Sci. 46:65-85.

Salmond GC, Geddes MK, Salmond CE. 1977. The Health of Former Servicemen. War Pensions Medical Research Trust Board, Wellington, New Zealand.

Speed N, Engdahl BE, Schwartz J, et al. 1989. Posttraumatic stress disorder as a consequence of the prisoner of war experience. J. Nerv. Ment. Dis. 177:147-153.

Strom A (ed.). 1968. Norwegian Concentration Camp Survivors. Oslo University Press, Oslo.

Sutker PB, Allain AN. 1991. MMPI profiles of veterans of WW II and Korea: comparisons of former POWs and combat survivors. Psychol. Rep. 68(1):279-284.

Sutker PB, Winstead DK, Galina ZH, Allain AN. 1990. Assessment of long-term psychosocial sequelae among POW survivors of the Korean conflict. J. Pers. Assess. 54(1&2):170-180.

Sutker PB, Winstead DK, Galina ZH, Allain AN. 1991. Cognitive deficits and psychopathology among former prisoners of war and combat veterans of the Korean conflict. Am. J. Psych. 148:67-72.

Tennant C, Goulston K, Dent O. 1986a. Clinical psychiatric illness in prisoners of war of the Japanese: forty years after release. Psychol. Med. 16:833-839.

Tennant C, Goulston K, Dent O. 1986b. The psychological effects of being a prisoner of war: forty years after release. Am. J. Psychiatry 143:618-621.

Thygesen P, Hermann K, Willanger R. 1970. Concentration camp survivors in Denmark: persecution, disease, disability, compensation. Dan. Med. Bull. 17:65-108.

Trimble MR. 1985. Post-traumatic stress disorder: history of a concept. In Figley CR (ed.), Trauma and Its Wake: The Study of Post-Traumatic Stress Disorder, Brunner/Mazel, New York.

Ursano RJ, Rundell JR. 1990. The prisoner of war. Mil. Med. 155:176-180.

Wilson JD, Braunwald E, Isselbacher KJ, et al. 1991. Harrison's Principles of Internal Medicine, 12th ed. McGraw-Hill, Inc., New York.

Zeiss RA, Dickman HR. 1989. PTSD 40 years later: incidence and person-situation correlates in former POWs. J. Clin. Psychol. 45:80-87.

9

Future Work

Many reports of this kind end with a call for more research. The circumstances in this case, however, justify such a prompting. For despite the indications that a large amount of data has been collected and reported, more has been left undone than has been accomplished. This chapter outlines some of this remaining work in the hope that it will encourage future investigations.

First, some data have not been analyzed. It was noted earlier that POWs examined by the VA under its protocol program before this research began (the so-called volunteers) were reinvited for a second examination. A number of volunteers had a second exam, but because only one examination per subject was analyzed in this report (generally, the last exam), some earlier examination material remains unanalyzed. In particular, for the selected group of twice-examined volunteers, it is possible to compare the results of the first and second examinations; such a comparison should provide interesting information on examination variability. Along the same lines, unbeknownst to the coding contractor, a small number of examinations were submitted for coding a second time. A comparison of the two codings of the same exam would provide useful information on the completeness and accuracy of the coding process.

Other kinds of data are also available. All operations and surgical procedures have been abstracted, coded, and computerized, but have not yet been analyzed. In addition, for each medical condition, all associated medications were listed and keyed, but not coded. Both these procedural and medication data might be expected to shed additional light on selected topics. For example, the Australian findings that showed an increased history of ulcer were confirmed by supplemental data on the use of cimetidine, and a possible increase in the prevalence of arthritis was suggested by increased use of analgesics.

Second, further analyses of the examination data could be undertaken to broaden the preliminary results presented in this report. For example, evidence was presented comparing the examination diagnosis of posttraumatic stress disorder (PTSD) with the Structured Clinical Interview for DSM-III-R (SCID) and the Mississippi scale diagnoses. Data are available for item-by-item analyses of the SCID and Mississippi questionnaires to determine which items are most strongly correlated with the clinical diagnosis of PTSD. Also of interest would be a comparison of lifetime and current PTSD prevalences, given that there was little difference between the two physician-based estimates and a sizable difference for the SCID. Because a diagnosis of PTSD is based on the meeting of four criteria, an examination of changes over time in criterion scores could provide an unparalleled opportunity to study the natural history of PTSD over several decades. In addition, those subjects who met some but not all criteria ("partial PTSD") could be profitably studied. Along more strictly methodological lines, a sample of the examinations could be reassessed by an outside panel to estimate interexaminer or even interhospital variability in the diagnosis of PTSD.

The psychological data from several sources might also be profitably compared and combined to gain more insight into psychiatric illnesses. A comparison of PTSD and depressive symptoms, for example, would provide important data on the comorbidity, or joint occurrence, of these two diagnoses. For another example, a discriminant analysis might be done, using all the psychiatric data, to compare POWs versus controls or even one POW group with another. Such an analysis could help determine which psychiatric scales or items distinguish subjects with PTSD from those without it by studying these relationships in one random half-sample and validating them in the other. It should also be noted that analyses like those of Chapter 6, which link examination conditions and prison camp treatment, did not include any demographic factors, although such an addition could provide further useful information. Similar analyses (with or without demographic factors) could be done using the SCID and questionnaire-derived measures of psychiatric illness.

Third, perhaps the most potentially fruitful area of secondary analysis (i.e., that would not require the collection of additional data) involves the linkage of previously and currently collected data. For example, the 1984–1985 questionnaire survey included the Center for Epidemiologic Studies depression (CES-D) scale, thus making it possible to compare 1984–1985 CES-D scores with current scores. Because the course of depressive symptoms is known to vary, this kind of test-retest analysis should provide useful information on the variability of depressive symptoms among POWs. Even the so-called lifetime prevalence data, based on the results of a single exam, could be refined and expanded by supplementing exam findings with earlier data from questionnaires and records to obtain a more complete, accurate measure of lifetime prevalence.

Closely related to these kinds of analyses are longitudinal studies that would link data collected earlier to subsequent outcomes. One example is the use of 1984–1985 data on depressive symptoms, together with demographic data on such factors as age and education, to predict PTSD rates in the current examination. Including some of the 1967 data from the Cornell Medical Index as well as even earlier hospitalization data (although cumulative response rates could be a problem) would permit an analysis linking five decades worth of information—a unique opportunity to explicate the processes by which such diseases progress.

Of course, a study such as this one always suggests new data that might be collected, but the disappointingly low response rates for this exam make new data collection even more important. New studies focused on a narrower clinical area and smaller and perhaps less geographically dispersed groups should have a better chance of achieving high response rates—the nerve conduction studies done by Hong at the Livermore VA Medical Center offer an example. If such efforts were to be mounted using a sample of the current respondents from the MFUA survey, any new clinical findings could be related to the examination data that have already been collected as well as to risk factor data in earlier questionnaires and records. The conditions in Table 6.7 would be obvious candidates for small-scale clinical studies, but others could also be profitably studied. The detailed diagnostic tabulations in Appendix C, which are described in Chapter 8, are provided as reference material to guide such investigations.

Finally, it has been approximately 15 years since the last mortality follow-up was completed. There is considerable speculation about current death rates among POWs but no comprehensive data. Although conditions like peripheral neuropathy and osteoarthritis can only be studied reasonably as morbid conditions, other conditions can be better investigated by using mortality data. An important point in favor of mortality studies—especially given the low response rates confronted in this study—is the completeness of death reporting, customarily 90% or better. The analyses of Chapter 6 suggest that simple comparisons of POWs and controls may not be as powerful a mechanism to identify associations with military captivity as are explicit analyses of the associations between health outcomes and prison camp factors. To date, the mortality analyses of the MFUA cohort have not attempted to associate mortality rates directly with prison camp factors. Such analyses could be undertaken and, with an additional 15–20 years of mortality data, might uncover further unsuspected links between the POW experience and subsequent medical conditions.

APPENDIXES

A

VA Circulars

This appendix includes the text of the first two VA Circulars published for this study. The first VA Circular, 10-87-138, was published in December 1987 and dealt with the examination of only POWs. It is here included without the Structured Clinical Interview for DSM-III-R (SCID) form. The second VA Circular, 10-88-117, was published in October 1988 and dealt only with the examination of non-POW veteran controls. A later VA Circular, 10-90-070, published in June 1990, superseded these earlier two circulars, but it is essentially a compilation of the earlier two and thus is not included here.

Single copies of the SCID and the psychological forms (VA Forms 10-20844-a through 10-20844-d) are available from the author.

Veterans Administration
Department of Medicine and Surgery
Washington, DC 20420

CIRCULAR 10-87-138

November 20, 1987

TO: Regional Directors; Medical District Directors; Directors, VA Medical Center Activities, Domiciliary, Outpatient Clinics and Regional Offices with Outpatient Clinics

SUBJ: Research Study of Former Prisoners of War

1. PURPOSE: The purpose of this Circular is to outline the methodology necessary to conduct a research study involving former POWs (prisoners of war).

2. POLICY: The Veterans Administration Office of Research and Development has contracted with the NAS-NRC (National Academy of Sciences-National Research Council) to conduct a research study focused on the long-term health effects of imprisonment as a POW. While Circular 10-85-48 outlines a standard evaluation of these veterans, additional steps are necessary to conduct the research study.

3. DISCUSSION:

a. It has been estimated that approximately 80,000 former Prisoners of War (POWs) from World War II and the Korean conflict are still living. Studies in this country and abroad have shown that the physical deprivation and psychological stress endured as a captive have lifelong effects on subsequent health and social adjustment. For example, specific residual health effects are known to be caused by prior malnutrition. In general, former POWs have significantly higher incidence rates for illnesses in many body systems, more frequent periods of hospitalization, and longer hospital stays. Vulnerability to psychological stress is also markedly increased.

b. The NAS-NRC is currently conducting, under VA contract, a morbidity survey of former prisoners of war of WW II and the Korean conflict, continuing an ongoing longitudinal study begun in the early 1950's. Their current study is designed to collect information from the existing DM&S POW protocol examination (including history, physical examination, mental status examination, and social work survey) and add it to other existing data. The general outline of the study is simple. The NAS-NRC will invite the veterans in their national sample who have not already been examined to undergo the DM&S POW protocol examination. When the examination is completed, a copy of the results will be sent to VA Central Office for coding and abstracting by the NAS-NRC. These new POW protocol examination data will be added to earlier NAS-NRC data to be analyzed together, and the results will be published.

c. The DM&S POW protocol examination program was begun in response to Pub.L. 97-37, the "Former Prisoners of War Benefits Act of 1981", when it was anticipated that many former POWs would contact the Veterans Administration to determine their eligibility under this law. Accordingly, DM&S developed a standard medical evaluation protocol. In order to adapt this program for research purposes, it is necessary to collect protocol examination data on representative groups of former POWs rather than to analyze data for only men who have presented themselves for examination. A later circular will address the examination of a control group of non-POW veterans to which comparisons can be made.

d. The NAS-NRC study group contains a sample of former POWs who have been carefully selected to be representative of all WW II and Korean conflict POWs. Because of this design, sound inferences can be made from these samples to

CIRCULAR 10-87-138
November 20, 1987

the group of all POWs. There are approximately 2,000 POWs in the NAS-NRC study, and most medical centers should expect to examine not more than 10-15 of them.

4. ACTION:

a. General Outline of the Research Study:

(1) The NAS-NRC will contact their research veterans and invite them to participate in the VA's protocol examination program, which has OMB approval number 29-0389. If a veteran agrees to be examined, a copy of the veteran's reply form will be sent to the nearest VA medical center. This reply form will contain the veteran's name, address, and telephone number(s) which can be used to contact the veteran for examination scheduling. The individual reply forms for each VAMC will be accompanied by a list (NAS-NRC POW Examination Schedule List.) This list will contain the veteran's name, Social Security number, and the NAS-NRC case number (study identification number), and POW status (POW in all cases), as well as room for entering a "status code" (described below) and the date the examination has been scheduled. The list will serve as a control list so that each VAMC knows which veterans are to be scheduled for examination and which have already been scheduled. It is possible that a VAMC will be sent more than one list as more veterans decide to come in for examination. Each of these lists should be processed independently.

(2) When the veteran is contacted for examination, one of the following codes (status codes) should be entered on the NAS-NRC Schedule List:

Code	Interpretation
1	Exam scheduled (also enter date of exam on list)
2	Exam previously done (do not repeat unless previous exam was incomplete)
3	Unable to contact (e.g., wrong telephone number)
4	Veteran refused examination (changed mind)
5	Veteran physically unable to come for exam
6	Veteran deceased
7	Able to contact, but veteran moved out of area or at another VAMC (specify)

(a sample NAS-NRC schedule list is in Attachment A)

(3) After the examination is scheduled, a copy of VA form 10-0048 should be sent to the veteran along with a study consent form (Attachment B), the standard VA research consent form (VA form 10-1086), and the usual cover letter (Attachment C). If in contacting the veteran, you find that the veteran has already been examined under the POW protocol and the previous examination was complete, do not bring the veteran in for a repeat examination. Instead, use code 2 above and send in a copy of the already completed exam, if it is available. If the previous exam was at a different VAMC, use code 7 and write the name of that VAMC in the schedule list margin.

(4) When the scheduling for all the veterans on a particular list has been completed, that list should be returned to VA Central Office. When the examinations themselves are completed, copies of the complete examination packages, including VA forms 10-0048, should be sent to the VA Central Office

CIRCULAR 10-87-138
November 20, 1987

addressee given on page 4 of this circular within 30 days after completion of the examination. Examinations should be sent in individually as they are completed, rather than being held and mailed in a group.

(5) The designated VA medical center POW physician coordinator will serve as principal investigator at VA Medical Center. The physician coordinator will be the contact person regarding this research project, and will assist the VA medical center's Research and Development Committee in obtaining the Subcommittee on Human Studies approval.

(6) The designated VA medical center POW administrative coordinator will coordinate the scheduling of examinations for the study participants and all other administrative aspects of the local study, such as ensuring that the Schedule List (paragraphs 4a.(1), (2), and (3)) is properly filled out and returned.

(7) Once the examinations are scheduled and the Schedule List returned, the POWs should be added to the DM&S POW Tracking System. This will allow the NAS-NRC to use the DM&S POW tracking system to follow the course of the examinations. Thus, it should not normally be necessary for the NAS-NRC to contact the VA medical center for status reports.

b. Conduct of Former POW Protocol Examination:

(1) When the veteran appears for examination, the POW administrative coordinator will explain the study. The short write-up in Attachment D ("What to Expect") should be copied and given to the veteran. At this time, the Informed Consent form (Attachment B) should be reviewed by the administrative coordinator, if it has not been mailed in beforehand, and the VA Form 10-0048 should be collected. The Informed Consent form should also be signed by the physician coordinator and witnessed, and a physician's progress note should accompany the Informed Consent form.

(2) The examination for NAS-NRC research veterans will be identical to the customary examination as set forth in DM&S Circular 10-85-48, with the following special emphases. Duodenal ulcer has been documented as a medical condition with higher prevalence among Australian former POWs; thus, a careful and detailed history of gastrointestinal problems must be taken. Of additional interest is the fact that these findings were substantiated by a higher prevalence of the use of cimetidine among former Australian POWs. Therefore, a careful medication history should also be included in the POW protocol examination. Data from the same Australian study further suggest that arthritis and the medications associated with arthritis may also appear at a higher rate in former POWs, and this should thus receive special emphasis in the examination.

(3) Psychological after-effects of military captivity may also persist among former POWs. For this reason, the required psychiatric consultation must be as thorough as possible and will include the structured clinical interview found in Attachment E.

(5) The NAS-NRC has agreed to reimburse examinees for their travel. When the examination has been completed the examinee should be given a copy of the "NAS-NRC Travel Reimbursement Request" (Attachment F) to be filled out while at

the VA medical center and mailed to the NAS-NRC. The NAS-NRC will handle all details of reimbursement after the travel requests have been received. Mail these requests to:

Mrs. Martha Bohman
Medical Follow-up Agency
National Research Council
2101 Constitution Ave.,N.W.
Washington, DC 20418.

(6) Each VA medical center will need to secure the approval of its local Research and Development Committee and Subcommittee on Human Studies. The VAMC physician coordinator will act as principal investigator for this purpose and will use the material in Attachment G in this process. Appendix G contains a protocol to be submitted, and Attachment B contains the Informed Consent form to be included in the package. The forms attached to this circular (10-20839a-d) may be reproduced locally as needed

(7) A conference call will be held to discuss this circular. Remaining general questions regarding this research study and the completed examination may be addressed to the following:

QUESTIONS TO:	FORMS TO:
Dr. William Page	Mr. David Thomas (151J)
Medical Follow-up Agency	Medical Research Service
National Research Council	VA Central Office
2101 Constitution Avenue,N.W.	810 Vermont Avenue, N.W.
Washington, DC 20418	Washington, DC 20420
FTS 737-2825	
Commercial 202-334-2825	FTS 373-3939

5. <u>REFERENCES</u>: None

6. <u>RESCISSIONS</u>: This DM&S Circular will be rescinded on November 18, 1988.

7. <u>FOLLOW-UP RESPONSIBILITY</u>: Assistant Chief Medical Director for Research and Development (151).

(signed)
ARTHUR J. LEWIS, M.D.
Deputy Chief Medical Director

Attachments

Distribution: COA: (10) only
SS (151F) FLD: RD, MDD, MA, DO, OC &
OCRO-1 plus 200-2
EX: Boxes 44-6 & 88-2,
Boxes 104, 60, 54, 52-1 each & 63-5

ATTACHMENT A

CIRCULAR 10-87-138
November 20, 1987

SAMPLE NAS-NRC POW EXAMINATION SCHEDULE LIST

FACILITY NAME AND NUMBER

VAMC Anywhere, 100

NAS-NRC CASE NUMBER	POW?	NAME	SSN	STATUS	DATE SCHEDULED
123456	Yes	veteran #1	123-45-6789	1	2/22/87
123457	Yes	veteran #2	123-45-6780	4	refusal
132456	Yes	veteran #3	231-54-9876	3	can't contact

ATTACHMENT B

CIRCULAR 10-87-138
November 20, 1987

INFORMED CONSENT

I ______________________________ a former prisoner of war or combat soldier, have been asked by Dr. ____
of ____VA Medical Center
to participate in an approved research project entitled "Medical Examination of Former Prisoners of War and Combat Soldiers." This study is being conducted by the Medical Follow-up Agency of the National Academy of Sciences-National Research Council under contract to the Veterans Administration.

1. I understand that this study will compare the physical health of former prisoners of war and combat soldiers, and that my physical health will be determined by medical examination.

2. The medical examination I will undergo will include a complete history and physical examination. There will also be a mental status evaluation, a social work survey, and psychological testing which will involve filling out forms with paper and pencil. There may be laboratory tests, as required, as a part of this examination. All medical results will be kept confidential. Information may be disclosed outside the VA only as permitted by the Privacy Act and other Federal laws.

3. I understand that my participation in this study might benefit me by providing a thorough medical examination, and that the study itself may benefit former prisoners of war and combat soldiers by helping to understand the effects of military service on health.

4. If I would prefer not to participate in this study or if I choose at any time to pull out of the study, I understand that I will continue to get the medical care I am eligible for under the rules of the VA. I understand that the results of this examination will be included in my VA medical record and that a copy of these results will be sent to the Medical Follow-up Agency of the National Academy of Sciences-National Research Council for their use in this scientific study. The Follow-up Agency is bound by the provisions of the Federal Privacy Act, and will not release any personal information about me to anyone. If I have any questions during or after this examination, I may call my VA doctor at

______________________________.

5. I have read or have had read to me all of the above and have received satisfactory explanation of the nature and purpose of the study. Any questions I have asked concerning this study have been answered to my satisfaction. I have also examined and signed VA Form 10-1086, Agreement to Participate in Research By or Under the Direction of the VA, which deals with further information I may need as a research volunteer.

I hereby consent to participate in this study.

______________________________ ______________________________
PATIENT DATE PHYSICIAN DATE

____
WITNESS DATE

ATTACHMENT C

CIRCULAR 10-87-138
November 20, 1987

COVER LETTER TO ACCOMPANY VA FORM 10-0048, FORMER POW MEDICAL HISTORY

Thank you for agreeing to participate in the National Academy of Sciences-National Research Council's research study of former POW (prisoners of war) and combat soldiers. Attached to this letter is a former POW Medical History form which will be made a permanent part of your record. Please complete this form to the best of your ability, paying special attention to completeness of responses. However, if you find it difficult to answer any part of the questionnaire, you may leave it blank.

Non-POWs should complete only items 1 through 12, 14, 25, 29, 30 through 37, 39, 40, and 54 through 62, replacing "captivity" with "combat" and "repatriation" with "release from active duty." If you have any questions about these changes, your administrative coordinator can help you with the form.

For your convenience, we have mailed this form to your home where you have access to military and other documents which may prove helpful in filling it out.

Also, included is a copy of the Informed Consent form for you to read. You should bring this form with you when you come for examination.

Please bring the completed forms to this facility on the day scheduled for your medical examination, which is on ______________________

at ________ A.M./P.M. in room ______________.

Your administrative coordinator for this evaluation is ______________,

who may be contacted by calling ______________. Please call your coordinator for any assistance needed in completing the history form and to confirm the appointment for your examination.

Attachments

ATTACHMENT D

CIRCULAR 10-87-138
November 20, 1987

WHAT TO EXPECT

The medical examination you will undergo today is provided by this VA medical center as part of a National Academy of Sciences-National Research Council study of the health of former prisoners of war and combat soldiers. The examination will include a complete physical examination, by one or more doctors, including medical history and appropriate laboratory tests. The examining physician will explain the need for and use of these tests to you. You will also be seeing a social worker for an interview and a psychiatrist for a consultation. These examinations are an important part of the research study. Because there are several parts to this examination, it may be necessary for you to wait before proceeding to the next part.

If you have any questions about the examination, you should talk to your administrative coordinator,________________________________.

ATTACHMENT G

CIRCULAR 10-87-138
November 20, 1987

NAS-NRC Research Protocol

Medical Examination Survey of Former Prisoners of War
of World War II and the Korean Conflict

Background

The Medical Follow-up Agency of the NAS-NRC (National Academy of Sciences-National Research Council) is presently conducting a morbidity survey of former POWs (prisoners of war) of WW II (World War II) and the Korean conflict. This survey continues earlier NAS-NRC research begun in the 1950's, and its purpose is the collection of medical examination data on former POWs and controls. In this regard, it is the first NAS-NRC study to collect medical examination data simultaneously on all participants.

Purpose

The goal of the research proposed here is to gather and analyze medical examination information from former POWs and comparable controls. The study design links the NAS-NRC's ongoing POW research and the Veterans Administration's POW medical evaluation program in order to secure information most efficiently. In brief, (details will be discussed in the methodology section), the VA medical evaluation protocol includes complete physical and psychiatric examinations by qualified VA medical personnel. Of special interest is the face-to-face psychiatric interview, which will gather information complementary to the current NAS-NRC questionnaire.

The following specific issues are among those to be addressed by this research proposal:

(1) Will psychiatric morbidity, as ascertained by interview and psychological evaluation, be higher among former WW II PWP (Prisoners of War Pacific) than among their comparable non-prisoner controls? Will this also hold true for WW II PWE (Prisoners of War European) and PWK (Prisoners of War Korean conflict) when compared to their respective controls? Will psychiatric morbidity be higher among PWP and PWK than PWE, as observed in earlier studies?

(2) What differences, if any, will there be between psychiatric morbidity assessed by interviewer versus questionnaire? Will these differences help us better understand the results from (1)?

(3) How have illness levels changed over time? In particular, has the earlier differential between the PWP and PWK groups, on the one hand, and the PWE group, on the other, decreased with time?

(4) How do the physician-reported physical examination findings compare to the self-reported diagnoses, symptoms, and complaints from the 1984 questionnaire? Are some physical findings under-reported or over-reported, and do non-medical factors influence this reporting?

(5) Can any signs of distinctive abnormal physical findings be seen in the PWE veterans who were seriously malnourished at repatriation?

Methodology

Since March, 1983, the VA Department of Medicine and Surgery has been conducting medical evaluations under a protocol set in DM&S circular 10-85-48. This protocol provides both a standardized format for medical evaluation and a standardized format for collecting POW medical history, the latter including a detailed history of captivity, repatriation, and postwar adjustment. The present proposal is designed to make use of this existing data collection mechanism. It is

CIRCULAR 10-87-138
November 20, 1987

important to note here that the VA Advisory Committee on Former POWs has previously recommended that the information contained in the medical history and examinations noted above be collected and made available for research use.

To date, approximately 22,000 examinations have been performed under this protocol. Given a universe of roughly 80,000 former POWs, one can estimate that 500-600 men in the current NAS-NRC study group have already received this examination at some VA Medical Center. These 500-600 examinations will be sent to NAS-NRC for coding, abstracting, and tabulating, and the remaining portion of the NAS-NRC cohort will be examined and those results similarly processed. The advantage of this proposal lies in its use of the current NAS-NRC cohort, which has two notable properties: it was statistically sampled to be representative of WW II and Korean conflict POWs, and it includes comparable control groups. These two characteristics distinguish the NAS-NRC cohort from any self-selected sample of men who have presented themselves for examination and allow sound inferences and generalizations to be made from the study cohort to the whole population of former POWs. The following paragraphs outline the methodological process in more detail.

The NAS-NRC cohort has been matched against the VA's file of completed examinations, using SSN (Social Security number) and claim number. This matching produced a file of NAS-NRC study veterans who have already been examined by the VA, and this file was then used to produce a separate list of examinined POWs for each VA medical center. These lists have been sent to the VA medical centers, and because the POWs on these lists have already been examined, each VA medical center has only to send copies of their completed examination forms to NAS-NRC. NAS-NRC has already begun to abstract, code, and computerize the completed examinations it has received.

While the already completed examinations are being processed, work will begin on the remainder of the cohort. All three POW groups (WW II Pacific, WW II European, and Korean conflict) were traced for the earlier survey, and mailing addresses have been obtained for approximately 90 percent of them. Letters of invitation will be mailed to these veterans, urging participation in the VA medical evaluation protocol, and requesting the veteran's permission to forward their name to the closest VA medical center for scheduling of the actual examination. Table 1 shows the number of POWs and controls by theater and by examination status.

Because the examination of controls necessitates additional clearance from the Office of Management and Budget (OMB), this examination will be addressed in a separate circular. For completeness, however, the process of non-POW control examinations is briefly outlined here. When clearance to examine is obtained, NAS-NRC will begin tracing the WW II and Korean conflict controls. This tracing includes matching against the VA BIRLS file to ascertain mortality and to obtain SSN. With SSN the living controls can then be forwarded to IRS through NIOSH for address finding. Veterans who are not traced through IRS will be given to commercial tracing firms to locate. Located control veterans will then be mailed the same invitation as the earlier POWs. The progress of examinations in both groups will be tracked so that copies of examinations can be requested as soon as they have been completed; some site visits will be made to monitor examination processes.

As part of the medical evaluation process, both POWs and controls will be invited to undergo further psychological testing; when clearance form OMB is obtained, these psychological tests will be mailed to individuals and returned directly to the NAS-NRC. The psychological test battery will consist of the following: (1) the 21-item Beck Depression Inventory; (2) the 20-item Center for Epidemiologic Studies Depression Scale; (3) the 90-item Hopkins Symptom Checklist ; and (4) a post-traumatic stress disorder checklist.

CIRCULAR 10-87-138
November 20, 1987

The psychiatric consultation, part of the usual medical evaluation, has traditionally been unstructured, thus permitting great differences in the documentation and recording of clinical findings. For research purposes, a structured and more standardized clinical psychiatric assessment will be incorporated into the psychiatric consultation. This will be accomplished by including the post-traumatic stress disorder portion of the SCID-NP-V (Structured Clinical Interview for DSM-III-R, Non-patient Version), which is currently also being employed in a national study of Vietnam veterans and PTSD. Moreover, the SCID-NP-V is fully compatible with DSM-II-R, assuring a common framework for diagnosing and reporting psychiatric disorders. The incorporation of this portion of the SCID-NP-V into the customary psychiatric consultation thus provides an opportunity to "calibrate" the psychiatric examination, facilitating the comparison of results to ongoing and future studies.

Copies of all completed medical evaluations will be abstracted, coded, and computerized. All medical examination, psychological testing, and disability data will be matched to the NAS-NRC master file to create a study file containing medical examinations, psychological tests, VA hospitalization experience, VA disability history, military service history, and POW captivity history. The study file will be analyzed to address the questions posed earlier, and a report will be prepared and submitted for publication.

Discussion

In this section, we address some of the practical issues in the study as outlined. Based on current data, it appears that roughly one-quarter of the NAS-NRC POW cohort has already presented itself to the VA for the medical examination protocol; this is approximately the same percentage as in the universe of all POWs. Thus, there are already approximately 600 NAS-NRC study veterans examined. Because protocol examination rates appear to be declining with time it is not reasonable to simply wait for more study veterans to present themselves to the VA for examination.

Confounding factors play an important part in the analysis of the data from this epidemiological study. An advantage of the longitudinal data base provided by the NAS-NRC cohort is that many possible confounders of health and disability have been recorded: demographic data, such as age, race, marital status; military data, such as duration of service, rank, theater of service; and data from other sources, such as smoking and drinking behavior from the current questionnaire. These factors can be controlled in analysis when outcome measures are compared and when associations with other risk variables are calculated.

CIRCULAR 10-87-138
November 20, 1987

Table 1

Estimated Sample Sizes for POW Medical Examination Study

War period and theater	POWs Already examined	POWs To be examined	Total	CONTROLS
WW II, Pacific	175	475	650	700
WW II, European	95	280	375	385
WW II, European (malnourished)	60	190	250	-
Korean conflict	220	620	840	850
Total	550	1,565	2,115	1,935

Veterans Administration
Department of Medicine and Surgery
Washington, DC 20420

CIRCULAR 10-88-117

October 7, 1988

TO: Regional Directors; Medical District Directors; Directors, VA Medical Center Activities, Domiciliary, Outpatient Clinics and Regional Offices with Outpatient Clinics

SUBJ: Examination of Controls in the Research Study of Former Prisoners of War (OMB 2900-0427)

1. PURPOSE: The purpose of this Circular is to outline the methodology necessary to conduct examinations of non-prisoner of war veteran controls who are part of the research study of former POWs (prisoners of war). Because the research study is only a one-time study, this Circular will not be incorporated into the Research Manual (M-3).

2. POLICY: The Veterans Administration Office of Research and Development has contracted with the NAS-NRC (National Academy of Sciences-National Research Council) to conduct a research study focused on the long-term health effects of imprisonment as a POW. Circular 10-87-138 contained the methodology for examining POWs; this Circular discusses the examination of non-POW veteran controls.

3. DISCUSSION:

a. As noted in Circular 10-87-138, studies of former prisoners of war have shown that the physical deprivation and psychological stress endured as a captive have lifelong effects on subsequent health and social adjustment. A crucial part of the scientific design of such studies is the comparison of the health of former POWs to that of veterans of comparable service who were not POWs, that is, non-POW veteran controls.

b. The NAS-NRC is currently conducting, under VA contract, a morbidity survey of former prisoners of war of WW II and the Korean conflict, continuing an ongoing longitudinal study began in the early 1950's. The design of the study was outlined in Circular 10-87-138, and this Circular adds the examination of non-POW veteran controls to the study.

4. ACTION:

a. General Outline of the Research Study:

The NAS-NRC has already invited the POWs in their research study to participate in the DM&S POW protocol examination program, and they soon will also invite non-POW veteran controls to participate. Once these non-POW controls agree to participate, their reply form will be sent to the nearest VA medical center for examination scheduling, just as the reply forms for POWs were sent. All reply forms will be accompanied by the NAS-NRC POW Examination Schedule List, as described in Circular 10-87-138. All of the steps outlined in Circular 10-87-138, paragraph 4a.,(1) - (6) will apply to the examination of non-POW controls. Non-POW veteran controls should not, however, be added to the DM&S POW Tracking System.

b. Conduct of the Examination of Non-POW Veteran Controls

(1) The conduct of the examination of non-POW veteran controls will be identical, as much as possible, to the conduct of the examination of former POWs as outlined in Circular 10-87-138. The same examination processes should be

CIRCULAR 10-88-117
October 7, 1988

undertaken for non-POW controls, namely: physical examination, mental health evaluation (including the structured clinical interview for DSM-III-R in Attachment E of Circular 10-87-138), social work interview, and psychological testing (using VA Form 10-20844-a through d).

(2) The POW Medical History form, VA Form 10-0048, will be filled out only partially, as follows:

items 1-12 and 14, leaving out references to time of capture and time of repatriation;
items 29, 30-37, using experiences during <u>combat</u> rather than captivity;
items 39-42, again with <u>combat</u> replacing captivity; and
items 54-60 and 62, with <u>release from active military duty</u> replacing repatriation.

Copies of the completed examination package should be sent to the address listed below in paragraph (5).

(3) The NAS-NRC has agreed to reimburse examinees for their travel. When the examination has been completed the examinee should be given a copy of the "NAS-NRC Travel Reimbursement Request" (Attachment A) to be filled out while at the VA medical center and mailed to the NAS-NRC. The NAS-NRC will handle all details of reimbursement after the travel requests have been received. Mail these requests to

Medical Follow-up Agency
National Research Council
2101 Constitution Avenue, N.W.
Washington, DC 20418

(4) Each VA medical center will need to secure the approval of its local Research and Development Committee and Subcommittee on Human Studies. The material attached to VA Circular 10-87-138 may be used for this purpose, and it is permissible to combine the application for approval for examination of non-POW controls with the earlier application for examination of POWs.

(5) Questions concerning this Circular and completed examinations may be addressed to the following:

QUESTIONS TO:	FORMS TO:
Dr. William Page	Mr. David Thomas (151J)
Medical Follow-up Agency	Medical Research Service
National Research Council	VA Central Office
2101 Constitution Avenue, N.W.	810 Vermont Avenure, N.W.
Washington, DC 20418	Washington, DC 20420
FTS 737-2825	FTS 373-3939
Commercial 202-334-2825	

5. <u>REFERENCES</u>: VA Circular 10-87-138.

6. <u>RESCISSIONS</u>: This DM&S Circular will be rescinded on October 9, 1989.

CIRCULAR 10-88-117
October 7, 1988

7. <u>FOLLOW-UP RESPONSIBILITY</u>: Assistant Chief Medical Director for Research and Development (151).

(signed)
ARTHUR J. LEWIS, M.D.
Deputy Chief Medical Director

Attachments

DISTRIBUTION:	COA:	(10) only (101B2)-5
SS (151F)	FLD:	RD, MDD, MA, DO, OC & OCRO-1 plus 200-2
	EX:	Boxes 44-6 & 88-2, Boxes 104, 60, 54, 52-1 each & 63-5

ATTACHMENT A

CIRCULAR 10-88-117
October 7, 1988

NAS-NRC TRAVEL REIMBURSEMENT REQUEST

DATE:______________

NAME:____

ADDRESS:____

____

NAS-NRC Case number: ________________________

VA medical center name:__________________________

Number of trips made:_____________

Number of miles traveled per round trip:________ Under 5

________ 5-10

________ 11-20

________ 21-50

________ 51-100

________ More than 100

Mileage rate: 21 cents per mile up to $75.00 maximum per trip.

Minimum payment $5.00 per trip.

____
Traveler's signature (must be signed to receive reimbursement)

VA FORM 10-20877
AUG 1988

B

List of Site Visits to VA Medical Facilities (with Map)

Date	Sites
February 1987	Miami VAMC, Riviera Beach OPC, Tampa VAMC
February 1987	Loma Linda VAMC, West Los Angeles VAMC (Brentwood and Wadsworth divisions), Long Beach VAMC
June 1987	Boston OPC, Boston VAMC, Northampton VAMC
May 1988	Manhattan VAMC, Bronx VAMC, Brooklyn OPC, East Orange VAMC
June 1988	American Lake (Tacoma) VAMC
October 1988	Allen Park (Detroit) VAMC, Saginaw VAMC
December 1988	San Francisco VAMC, Palo Alto VAMC, Sacramento OPC
February 1989	Phoenix VAMC, Tucson VAMC
July 1989	Martinsburg VAMC
August 1989	Asheville VAMC
November 1989	Minneapolis VAMC
February 1990	Dallas VAMC, San Antonio VAMC
June 1990	Salt Lake City VAMC
January 1991	Albuquerque VAMC
June 1991	Buffalo VAMC
August 1991	Denver VAMC, Sheridan (Wyoming) VAMC, Miles City (Montana) VAMC

VAMC = Department of Veterans Affairs Medical Center; OPC = Outpatient Clinic.

POW Research Study
Site Visits* to VA Medical Centers

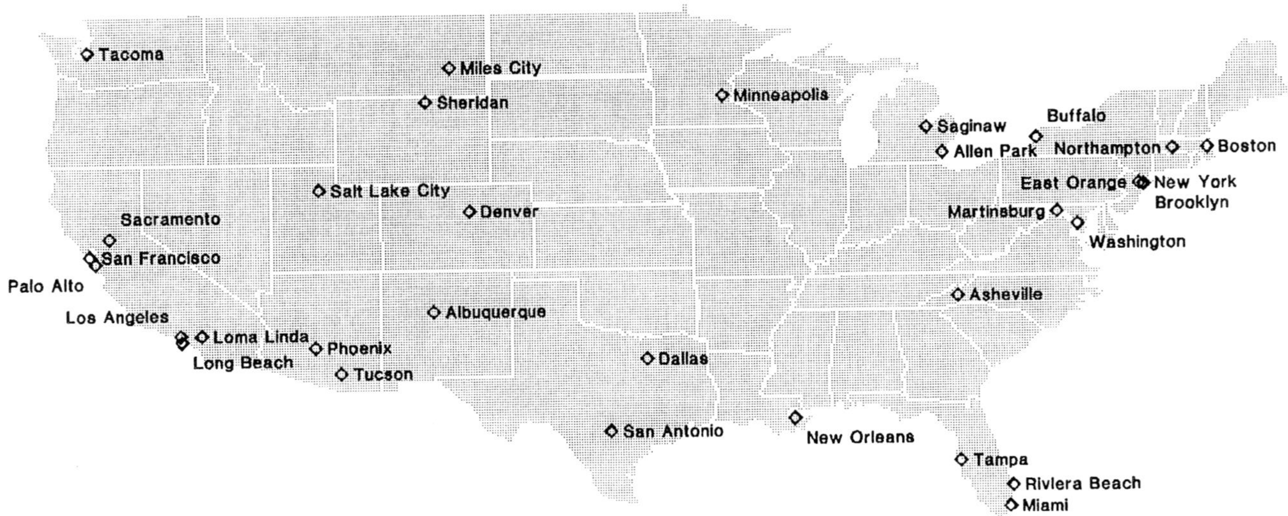

*Feb 1987 through August 1991

C

Detailed Diagnostic Data from the Medical Examination

This appendix contains detailed diagnostic data from the medical examination for each POW and control group studied. In contrast to the other tables in this report, however, the data in this appendix are not person-based counts—each mention of a particular condition is counted, even if it occurs many times for the same individual in different parts of a single examination. The data have been aggregated to the 3-digit ICD code level by truncating additional 4th and 5th digits.

GROUP=PWP

DIAG	Frequency
002	3
004	1
006	48
007	3
008	1
009	172
011	58
017	4
032	22
033	9
034	9
035	1
038	2
041	7
045	5
050	5
052	30
053	8
054	1
055	34
056	1
061	57
063	1
065	1
070	30
072	29
076	1
078	5
079	1
081	3
084	275
088	1
097	2
098	3
099	3
102	4
110	63
111	2
114	4
117	4
120	7
121	1
123	1
125	1
126	6
127	14
128	25
129	10
132	6
133	24
134	1
136	4
138	3
139	4
140	2
154	2
161	10
162	1
169	4
172	6
173	62
185	17
188	6
189	5
191	4
195	2
197	1
199	3
202	1
210	1
211	17
214	7
215	3
216	10
217	1
219	1
223	1
224	1
226	1
228	1
229	1
238	1
239	5
240	2
241	5
242	4
244	20
246	1
250	92
251	4
255	1
256	1
259	2
261	20
262	2
263	160
264	1
265	363
266	5
267	58
268	1
269	92
271	1
272	53
273	2
274	22
275	14
276	34
277	5
278	37
279	1
280	5
281	1
282	4
285	15
286	2
288	12
289	10
290	9
291	6
292	18
294	2
295	5
296	18
297	3
298	29
300	398
301	54
302	106
303	31
304	3
305	208
306	14
307	164
308	36
309	181
310	26
311	144
312	16
315	2
322	3
323	1
324	1
331	11
332	16
333	3
337	4
342	8
344	25
345	9
346	11
347	4
348	7
349	2
351	4
352	1
353	1
354	16
355	29
356	38
357	22
358	6
359	1
360	9
362	37
363	6
365	20
366	53

367	62	444	6	530	27
368	186	446	1	531	11
369	63	447	8	532	41
370	6	448	3	533	48
371	15	451	9	535	12
372	12	453	4	536	63
373	1	454	73	537	20
374	7	455	100	540	12
375	1	456	6	541	15
377	11	457	4	542	1
378	8	458	11	543	26
379	43	459	19	550	72
380	24	460	4	551	1
381	2	461	2	553	111
382	18	462	7	556	3
383	5	463	3	558	86
384	16	465	4	560	4
385	5	466	2	562	55
386	4	470	35	564	56
387	1	471	3	565	5
388	131	472	5	566	1
389	302	473	45	568	1
390	9	474	35	569	31
391	1	477	13	571	16
393	1	478	17	573	89
394	7	480	1	574	20
397	2	482	3	575	36
398	2	485	4	576	1
401	263	486	117	577	8
402	14	487	9	578	52
403	1	490	11	579	55
405	2	491	17	580	1
410	84	492	40	583	3
411	4	493	27	584	4
412	4	494	3	585	5
413	58	496	70	587	3
414	90	500	1	588	2
415	1	501	1	590	2
416	9	507	2	591	3
420	7	510	2	592	53
424	17	511	57	593	16
425	4	512	2	594	10
426	48	513	1	595	6
427	112	514	5	596	6
428	27	515	17	597	1
429	104	516	7	598	2
430	1	518	38	599	37
431	1	519	11	600	115
433	2	520	6	601	29
434	1	521	13	602	23
435	14	522	10	603	7
436	33	523	48	604	12
437	1	525	214	606	4
440	58	526	2	607	16
441	17	527	1	608	29
442	1	528	13	611	9
443	67	529	5	656	1

680	14	782	449	878	1
682	10	783	270	879	10
685	9	784	143	880	7
686	12	785	99	881	8
689	1	786	346	882	7
690	9	787	187	883	3
692	32	788	221	884	6
693	6	789	103	886	7
695	6	790	157	890	7
696	7	791	15	891	49
698	61	793	6	892	12
700	6	794	35	904	1
701	20	795	2	905	5
702	34	796	19	907	4
703	24	799	172	909	6
704	14	801	1	910	1
706	18	802	14	913	1
707	35	803	3	918	1
708	11	805	11	919	5
709	193	807	13	920	3
711	1	810	4	921	4
712	1	812	17	922	3
714	7	813	11	923	1
715	153	814	10	924	2
716	112	815	7	926	3
717	4	816	6	927	1
718	16	818	6	941	2
719	495	820	2	943	3
720	15	821	3	945	4
721	133	822	4	948	5
722	78	823	5	949	6
723	41	824	19	956	2
724	250	825	16	957	1
726	45	826	8	958	2
727	10	827	1	959	130
728	76	829	2	973	1
729	151	831	5	977	1
730	4	836	1	983	1
731	6	840	3	986	1
732	4	844	2	990	4
733	39	845	3	991	74
734	21	846	8	992	11
735	25	847	4	993	1
736	33	848	3	994	30
737	47	850	9	995	167
738	5	853	4	996	4
741	1	854	21	997	1
743	4	862	2	998	4
747	3	863	2	E800	1
751	4	866	3	E805	1
752	2	870	3	E807	1
755	2	871	2	E812	1
756	6	872	5	E816	4
757	1	873	22	E818	3
759	1	874	1	E819	13
780	770	875	6	E826	1
781	93	876	9	E828	1

E841	3
E844	1
E848	2
E849	15
E864	1
E878	1
E879	4
E884	3
E885	1
E887	3
E888	11
E898	1
E901	3
E912	2
E915	2
E916	8
E917	11
E919	1
E920	6
E922	1
E924	3
E926	2
E927	4
E928	15
E929	3
E930	14
E931	2
E934	1
E935	5
E937	1
E942	3
E943	1
E944	6
E946	1
E947	4
E958	1
E960	9
E966	2
E968	165
E988	1
E991	63
E993	13
E994	3
E995	13
E996	1
E997	1
E999	1
V10	3
V16	64
V17	125
V18	31
V19	9
V25	1
V43	6
V44	4
V45	10
V57	1

V62	4

GROUP = PWEM

DIAG	Frequency
002	2
005	1
006	7
007	1
009	48
011	13
032	11
033	2
034	6
038	1
041	3
052	16
053	8
055	16
070	5
072	16
075	1
078	1
084	1
099	2
101	1
110	24
117	5
128	1
132	10
133	3
153	8
157	1
162	4
173	10
185	9
186	4
188	5
198	1
204	1
211	12
214	5
222	1
226	1
228	4
229	5
236	1
239	3
244	3
250	25
252	1
253	2
259	4
260	1
261	7
263	73
265	12
267	1
269	22

272	39	379	9	486	33
273	1	380	12	487	2
274	19	382	8	489	1
275	7	383	1	490	7
276	11	384	7	491	7
277	2	386	3	492	16
278	40	387	1	493	4
282	4	388	57	494	3
285	2	389	141	496	21
288	2	390	5	511	10
289	2	393	1	514	1
290	3	401	106	515	9
291	1	402	6	518	10
292	11	403	1	519	2
295	4	409	1	520	1
296	6	410	67	521	7
297	1	412	3	522	1
298	6	413	15	523	19
300	175	414	36	525	84
301	28	415	2	527	5
302	25	416	1	528	1
303	14	424	6	530	18
305	83	425	1	531	2
306	4	426	13	532	24
307	71	427	39	533	25
308	16	428	2	535	8
309	41	429	39	536	48
310	6	433	1	537	12
311	56	435	6	541	6
312	2	436	27	543	11
322	1	438	3	550	23
331	1	440	10	553	54
332	3	442	1	558	58
333	2	443	17	559	1
342	2	444	1	562	25
344	4	446	1	564	27
352	3	447	1	565	1
354	9	448	5	567	1
355	6	451	4	569	12
356	6	453	1	570	1
357	1	454	16	573	21
359	3	455	41	574	10
360	4	456	2	575	12
361	4	458	1	578	14
362	17	459	12	579	19
363	2	460	2	583	2
365	2	462	1	586	5
366	12	463	2	590	4
367	31	466	1	591	1
368	55	470	8	592	11
369	23	471	1	594	2
371	10	473	20	595	3
372	3	474	15	596	2
373	5	477	20	599	8
374	4	478	6	600	56
375	1	480	1	601	1
378	2	485	2	602	5

603	2
604	1
607	2
608	5
609	2
611	2
623	1
624	1
680	5
681	1
682	5
685	2
686	4
690	1
692	8
693	2
695	5
697	1
698	10
700	1
701	4
702	2
703	8
704	6
706	6
707	1
709	84
715	79
716	48
717	2
718	10
719	185
720	4
721	47
722	35
723	17
724	83
726	10
727	13
728	33
729	67
733	2
734	7
735	10
736	6
737	12
738	2
743	1
752	1
754	1
756	1
757	1
759	2
780	212
781	44
782	124
783	99
784	59
785	35
786	117
787	84
788	71
789	58
790	62
791	5
794	24
796	4
799	80
802	4
803	6
807	3
810	6
813	1
814	1
815	1
816	5
818	2
821	1
822	2
823	3
824	2
825	1
826	1
827	1
836	2
840	2
844	2
845	2
846	4
847	5
848	1
850	1
854	3
861	1
871	2
873	13
875	2
876	11
877	8
879	2
880	13
881	11
882	6
883	5
884	6
890	7
891	16
892	2
893	2
894	2
907	1
908	1
916	1
919	1
922	1
923	2
941	4
943	3
944	1
945	3
948	1
955	2
956	1
959	56
989	1
991	132
994	20
995	45
997	4
998	2
E819	4
E825	2
E826	1
E841	2
E844	1
E849	3
E860	1
E881	1
E882	1
E884	1
E885	1
E888	1
E904	1
E916	3
E919	2
E921	2
E928	2
E930	8
E933	1
E935	4
E944	1
E946	1
E960	2
E968	31
E990	1
E991	44
E993	3
E994	7
E995	1
V01	1
V12	3
V16	22
V17	55
V18	9
V19	6
V40	2
V45	13
V62	2

GROUP=PWE

DIAG	Frequency
002	2
006	12
009	55
011	3
018	1
032	1
033	6
034	6
038	2
041	9
052	20
053	2
055	29
056	1
070	3
072	25
078	6
084	6
098	1
099	4
110	22
111	2
112	2
115	4
117	2
132	5
133	5
136	3
141	2
142	10
153	15
154	8
161	2
172	2
173	21
175	2
185	13
189	2
195	1
198	1
199	3
211	15
213	3
214	11
215	3
216	8
229	3
232	1
238	3
239	6
240	1
242	2
244	19
246	2
250	53
251	5
252	2
259	1
263	56
265	4
269	18
271	1
272	48
274	15
275	10
276	26
277	7
278	17
281	5
282	1
285	10
288	7
289	1
291	2
292	19
295	2
296	2
297	2
298	3
300	197
301	15
302	44
303	12
305	186
306	16
307	74
308	19
309	62
310	10
311	84
312	2
320	2
323	1
331	3
333	3
335	1
336	1
342	12
344	5
345	2
346	8
350	2
351	3
353	2
354	5
355	7
356	2
357	3
360	5
361	8
362	17
363	2
364	1
365	7
366	58
367	29
368	108
369	17
371	8
372	6
373	2
374	3
375	1
377	1
378	1
379	21
380	5
382	5
383	1
384	6
385	3
386	2
388	70
389	197
390	10
391	2
394	2
396	1
398	1
401	158
402	7
410	78
411	1
413	32
414	44
416	1
423	4
424	5
425	1
426	32
427	97
428	7
429	53
433	1
434	1
435	13
436	21
437	1
440	23
441	4
443	19
444	1
447	2
448	1
451	5
453	1
454	37
455	70

456	4	553	56	720	9
457	1	556	3	721	69
459	11	558	57	722	57
460	5	560	1	723	16
462	3	562	30	724	161
463	1	564	42	726	16
464	2	565	5	727	19
465	3	567	6	728	31
466	1	569	20	729	83
470	19	571	2	730	2
471	7	573	19	731	2
472	12	574	4	733	11
473	43	575	22	734	2
474	33	577	1	735	11
476	1	578	32	736	32
477	8	579	27	737	17
478	23	583	5	738	7
485	1	584	3	741	2
486	43	586	4	746	1
487	4	592	23	747	1
490	3	593	5	748	1
491	7	594	3	750	3
492	21	596	3	752	2
493	27	599	14	754	3
496	39	600	70	780	320
498	1	601	3	781	49
500	1	602	19	782	153
501	1	603	7	783	175
502	1	607	15	784	76
507	1	608	12	785	79
511	22	611	8	786	169
512	2	680	2	787	87
515	19	684	1	788	112
516	1	685	2	789	55
518	29	686	12	790	131
519	7	690	10	791	11
520	1	692	15	792	2
521	14	693	6	793	1
522	3	695	7	794	38
523	32	696	5	796	6
524	1	697	4	799	120
525	109	698	24	802	12
527	2	700	1	803	1
528	2	701	14	805	6
529	3	702	14	807	10
530	21	703	8	812	12
531	11	704	11	813	4
532	20	706	13	814	7
533	40	707	3	815	9
535	15	708	5	816	6
536	67	709	107	818	2
537	10	714	14	820	5
540	4	715	121	821	1
541	10	716	74	822	3
543	26	717	2	823	5
544	1	718	7	824	5
550	55	719	359	825	6

826	1
827	5
831	5
836	5
840	6
842	2
844	3
845	7
846	6
847	3
850	3
853	3
854	10
863	1
868	1
871	8
872	4
873	17
874	1
875	5
877	4
878	1
879	18
880	9
881	5
882	7
883	3
884	3
886	13
890	15
891	49
892	3
906	1
909	1
910	1
911	1
916	1
917	2
919	3
920	1
922	1
924	6
928	1
941	17
942	2
943	4
944	5
945	2
948	9
949	2
950	7
951	1
958	1
959	90
991	94
994	23
995	49
996	1
998	1
999	1
E812	1
E814	1
E819	11
E844	2
E849	7
E878	1
E880	1
E881	2
E884	4
E885	2
E888	8
E898	1
E899	1
E901	1
E906	5
E914	3
E917	5
E919	4
E920	4
E922	5
E927	4
E928	4
E930	19
E931	1
E932	1
E935	5
E938	2
E942	6
E946	3
E960	9
E968	31
E991	79
E993	10
E994	48
E995	1
E998	1
V16	44
V17	91
V18	11
V19	13
V43	1
V44	5
V45	8
V62	1

GROUP = PWK

Diag.	Frequency
001	1
005	1
006	43
009	251
011	83
032	5
033	19
034	19
038	3
039	1
041	2
045	4
050	2
052	58
053	6
054	2
055	70
056	3
070	36
072	71
078	18
084	164
087	2
091	2
097	5
098	12
099	8
101	2
110	122
111	2
114	2
117	3
120	3
123	5
126	2
127	28
128	66
129	17
132	35
133	27
134	4
136	19
137	1
146	1
149	4
153	4
154	14
161	11
162	9
170	2
171	1
173	44
185	9
188	5
195	4
198	2
201	1
202	1
210	3
211	25
213	5
214	25
215	2
216	20
222	4
224	1
227	11
228	4
229	3
230	1
234	1
235	3
238	6
239	24
240	12
241	1
242	3
244	7
246	1
250	151
251	7
253	2
259	4
261	22
263	204
264	3
265	238
267	13
269	131
271	1
272	124
273	1
274	23
275	22
276	58
277	12
278	86
280	4
282	5
285	14
288	31
289	12
290	3
291	8
292	63
293	2
294	2
295	32
296	19
297	9
298	34
300	871
301	197
302	140
303	59
304	1
305	674
306	31
307	381
308	58
309	339
310	23
311	354
312	32
316	1
323	3
330	1
331	14
333	3
336	3
337	5
342	9
344	30
345	10
346	25
347	4
348	3
349	2
351	4
353	1
354	26
355	25
356	25
357	19
359	1
360	12
361	2
362	44
363	3
364	11
365	51
366	71
367	148
368	399
369	79
370	4
371	12
372	39
373	9
374	10
375	6
377	16
378	1
379	87
380	35
381	5
382	25
383	2

384	20	474	70	573	124
385	7	475	1	574	15
386	9	477	20	575	30
388	261	478	64	576	1
389	584	480	1	577	9
390	22	482	1	578	103
391	3	486	197	579	73
395	4	487	5	582	2
398	1	490	17	583	3
401	412	491	27	585	1
402	12	492	41	588	1
409	2	493	35	590	9
410	138	494	3	591	5
411	1	495	1	592	116
412	1	496	91	593	9
413	48	500	3	594	1
414	80	501	3	595	3
415	4	511	57	596	9
416	2	512	7	597	3
423	6	514	2	598	7
424	21	515	36	599	95
425	4	516	7	600	113
426	63	518	72	601	39
427	180	519	11	602	16
428	16	520	1	603	14
429	100	521	54	604	9
432	3	522	14	605	1
433	13	523	150	606	6
434	18	524	2	607	14
435	3	525	410	608	54
436	22	526	1	611	13
437	6	527	5	680	17
438	2	528	35	682	12
440	45	529	15	685	10
441	3	530	61	686	7
443	82	531	37	690	11
444	9	532	71	691	1
447	17	533	127	692	41
448	5	535	43	693	3
451	16	536	214	695	9
453	3	537	50	696	11
454	49	540	4	697	2
455	253	541	23	698	107
456	6	543	65	700	20
458	3	550	88	701	48
459	25	553	149	702	30
460	12	555	5	703	29
461	2	558	227	704	18
462	12	560	4	705	5
463	9	562	55	706	43
464	1	564	118	707	17
465	9	565	16	708	9
466	1	566	1	709	406
470	51	567	3	710	1
471	5	568	4	712	4
472	14	569	50	714	25
473	81	571	18	715	292

716	247	802	31	891	205
717	20	803	4	892	60
718	41	805	15	895	2
719	1226	807	34	901	1
720	45	808	2	904	1
721	257	810	14	905	4
722	122	812	20	906	1
723	83	813	9	909	5
724	530	814	19	910	1
725	1	815	14	911	1
726	87	816	13	912	1
727	21	818	6	913	1
728	153	820	4	914	3
729	350	821	21	917	1
730	19	822	6	919	2
731	2	823	17	920	2
732	4	824	23	921	5
733	35	825	19	922	2
734	18	826	3	924	4
735	50	827	6	927	6
736	68	829	3	928	2
737	60	831	8	930	1
738	26	833	1	935	1
740	1	834	1	940	2
743	1	835	3	942	3
748	1	836	4	943	5
749	2	837	1	944	3
750	2	839	7	945	13
751	2	840	7	948	8
752	2	841	1	949	2
753	6	842	3	951	4
754	4	844	6	952	2
755	1	845	23	956	4
756	4	846	18	957	2
757	2	847	20	959	239
758	3	850	29	977	2
759	4	851	1	984	1
768	1	854	43	986	1
780	1355	860	2	989	7
781	142	862	4	990	1
782	679	866	3	991	490
783	522	871	8	992	6
784	302	872	8	994	118
785	218	873	86	995	200
786	656	874	25	996	1
787	402	875	37	997	2
788	325	876	37	998	1
789	228	877	27	E812	4
790	342	879	50	E814	2
791	42	880	68	E816	3
792	3	881	49	E817	1
793	11	882	37	E818	1
794	87	883	10	E819	28
795	14	884	38	E822	1
796	36	885	2	E825	7
798	1	886	8	E832	1
799	467	890	90	E844	5

E849	20
E858	1
E862	1
E863	3
E864	1
E879	1
E881	6
E882	6
E883	2
E884	3
E885	10
E888	15
E900	2
E901	8
E905	1
E906	7
E916	11
E917	4
E918	2
E919	5
E920	10
E921	4
E922	5
E923	2
E924	4
E925	2
E927	21
E928	30
E929	3
E930	24
E931	3
E932	4
E933	1
E935	12
E936	1
E937	1
E941	1
E942	6
E943	1
E946	2
E947	3
E948	1
E949	1
E950	2
E952	1
E958	2
E960	23
E966	2
E968	215
E969	1
E980	3
E985	2
E991	372
E993	42
E995	27
E999	1
V10	3
V13	1
V16	106
V17	218
V18	55
V19	24
V43	2
V44	5
V45	4
V49	1
V62	3

GROUP=WP

DIAG	Frequency
006	1
007	2
009	4
032	3
033	4
034	3
049	3
052	5
053	1
054	1
055	8
056	1
061	7
070	2
072	4
078	2
084	59
098	2
110	24
114	1
117	5
162	3
173	9
188	8
197	5
211	8
214	9
216	3
228	1
239	2
240	2
244	6
250	24
263	1
272	30
274	2
275	9
276	19
277	3
278	8
282	1
285	13
288	3
292	2
296	3
298	1
300	18
302	14
303	9
305	87
306	1
307	10
308	1
309	5

311	13
312	1
324	4
336	1
342	1
344	2
354	3
355	3
356	1
357	2
361	2
362	5
365	4
366	29
367	12
368	38
369	6
371	2
373	1
374	1
379	2
380	9
382	6
383	1
384	5
388	32
389	76
390	2
401	41
410	26
413	12
414	23
415	3
423	1
424	2
426	15
427	16
428	2
429	14
436	4
440	10
441	3
443	11
447	4
448	2
451	2
454	11
455	24
459	2
460	1
462	5
464	2
470	8
471	3
473	6
474	9
477	3
478	4
480	5
485	1
486	12
490	6
491	2
492	18
493	5
496	12
511	4
513	1
515	3
516	1
518	7
519	3
521	5
523	3
525	32
530	5
531	7
532	6
533	7
535	2
536	5
537	2
541	3
543	13
550	29
553	11
557	1
558	10
562	4
564	5
565	1
569	10
571	3
573	14
574	6
575	6
578	4
579	4
590	1
592	11
593	2
594	1
596	2
599	4
600	37
601	5
602	15
603	4
607	2
608	10
611	7
680	2
682	2
692	2
696	2
698	9
701	4
702	7
703	5
704	4
706	4
707	2
708	2
709	50
711	1
714	5
715	36
716	15
718	1
719	64
720	1
721	36
722	22
723	8
724	41
726	9
727	1
728	6
729	21
730	1
733	4
734	4
735	4
736	2
737	9
738	5
757	2
759	1
780	57
781	5
782	46
783	15
784	19
785	11
786	44
787	17
788	36
789	5
790	70
791	10
793	1
794	30
796	5
798	1
799	10
802	6
803	1
805	5
807	5
810	2
812	2

813	1
814	2
816	1
818	2
820	3
825	1
827	1
831	1
846	2
847	2
850	2
854	4
871	1
872	1
873	4
874	5
875	5
876	5
880	7
881	1
882	6
883	2
884	4
890	6
891	8
892	6
893	2
894	2
910	1
918	1
921	1
959	24
991	3
994	1
995	17
998	2
E814	1
E819	3
E849	1
E854	1
E878	2
E881	2
E882	1
E885	1
E888	6
E916	3
E922	5
E930	8
E931	2
E935	1
E941	3
E944	2
E947	1
E960	2
E968	1
E991	21
E993	14
V16	14
V17	22
V18	10
V19	3
V62	1

GROUP=WE

DIAG	Frequency
006	1
009	1
034	1
052	1
053	1
055	2
070	3
072	2
079	2
084	3
097	2
099	1
135	1
173	14
188	2
195	3
211	1
214	1
216	2
239	2
242	1
250	8
271	1
272	15
274	2
275	3
276	11
277	1
278	1
285	3
288	1
291	4
300	3
302	8
303	8
304	2
305	28
307	5
308	1
309	5
312	2
336	1
355	1
356	1
360	2
364	1
365	4
366	15
367	3
368	12
369	1
379	4
380	7
382	1

384	1
388	2
389	27
401	30
410	5
413	1
414	1
424	2
426	6
427	18
429	6
440	6
443	1
444	1
447	1
448	1
451	1
454	3
455	5
456	1
459	1
460	1
465	1
470	2
473	2
474	6
477	1
478	3
486	11
490	1
492	3
496	6
515	4
518	3
521	2
523	8
524	1
525	15
530	1
531	1
532	1
533	2
536	2
537	1
543	6
550	8
553	11
558	1
562	3
565	1
569	2
573	2
578	1
579	4
592	12
593	1
599	1
600	7
602	1
603	3
607	1
678	1
686	1
690	1
692	1
695	1
698	5
701	2
702	2
703	1
706	1
709	18
715	11
716	11
719	43
720	2
721	7
722	9
724	19
726	3
728	6
729	7
733	2
734	2
736	2
737	2
738	2
756	1
780	25
781	7
782	16
783	4
784	7
785	9
786	19
787	6
788	14
789	1
790	34
791	3
793	1
794	10
795	1
796	2
799	3
805	2
807	1
813	1
824	1
825	1
827	1
836	2
840	2
854	3
875	1
880	2
881	2
882	3
886	3
890	2
921	1
923	1
941	1
944	1
959	9
990	1
991	8
995	4
E888	2
E904	1
E917	4
E919	1
E928	2
E930	2
E991	5
E993	1
E994	1
V16	9
V17	19
V18	3
V19	1

GROUP=WK

DIAG	Frequency
009	9
032	2
033	6
034	3
037	1
038	1
052	13
053	1
055	17
056	2
070	4
072	14
078	7
084	40
098	3
099	5
110	25
114	2
128	2
133	4
162	1
173	31
185	5
199	1
210	5
211	5
214	3
216	7
225	2
228	1
229	2
239	7
240	2
244	3
246	2
250	33
251	1
263	3
265	7
269	3
272	57
274	10
275	2
276	20
277	3
278	28
280	1
281	1
282	5
285	22
287	3
288	5
289	2
291	4
292	9
295	1
296	2
298	1
300	74
301	15
302	23
303	4
305	222
306	5
307	49
308	10
309	23
311	40
312	2
336	1
342	4
344	4
345	1
346	1
347	4
350	2
355	2
356	2
357	2
361	11
362	10
363	3
364	1
365	1
366	25
367	27
368	67
369	7
371	7
372	8
374	2
378	3
379	7
380	7
382	2
384	9
385	2
388	42
389	138
390	3
401	105
402	2
409	1
410	42
413	19
414	27
424	11
426	11
427	25
428	5
429	24
430	4
433	1
434	3
436	14
437	4
440	11
443	11
444	3
447	5
451	4
453	1
454	13
455	54
456	5
459	1
462	1
466	1
470	15
471	2
472	1
473	10
474	16
477	5
478	10
481	2
482	2
486	34
487	2
490	4
491	8
492	6
493	1
496	14
502	1
510	5
511	10
512	1
514	3
515	11
518	17
520	1
521	7
522	1
523	20
524	1
525	78
526	1
528	4
529	4
530	11
531	9
532	1
533	16
535	9
536	17
537	3
540	3

541	6
543	22
550	33
553	38
558	12
559	1
562	14
564	7
565	2
569	7
571	1
573	4
574	4
575	3
577	10
578	7
579	11
592	34
593	7
599	18
600	32
601	11
602	9
603	1
604	2
605	1
607	6
608	13
680	1
682	2
685	2
686	1
690	5
692	6
695	1
696	4
698	13
701	5
702	6
703	4
704	1
706	9
707	1
709	95
714	4
715	53
716	51
717	4
718	15
719	189
720	6
721	33
722	15
723	11
724	87
726	12
727	4
728	18
729	45
730	2
733	10
734	1
736	13
737	10
738	8
746	1
748	1
752	1
753	1
780	186
781	23
782	83
783	33
784	48
785	28
786	89
787	40
788	65
789	22
790	150
791	17
792	2
794	23
795	1
796	3
799	33
802	11
803	3
805	4
807	5
812	6
813	4
814	10
815	4
821	5
822	2
824	14
831	2
836	1
842	2
844	1
845	3
846	1
847	4
848	1
850	11
854	3
861	2
870	1
871	4
872	2
873	63
874	14
875	20
876	22
877	10
879	33
880	39
881	25
882	16
883	6
884	22
886	3
890	32
891	83
892	8
893	3
907	1
919	1
924	3
944	2
945	2
951	1
956	1
957	1
959	27
989	2
990	2
991	32
992	1
995	21
E812	4
E814	1
E819	7
E828	1
E849	13
E882	5
E884	2
E885	1
E886	3
E888	6
E900	1
E917	5
E919	1
E920	3
E924	3
E927	3
E928	6
E950	1
E968	4
E991	173
E992	1
E993	30
E994	3
V16	44
V17	64
V18	13
V19	12
V45	5
V49	1